Murray E. Allen, MD

Musculoskeletal Pain Emanating from the Head and Neck

Current Concepts in Diagnosis, Management and Cost Containment

Pre-publication
REVIEWS,
COMMENTARIES,
EVALUATIONS . . .

"**T**his is a good update on an important topic, useful text for general practitioners as well as for specialists who deal with musculoskeletal pain, particularly neck injuries. Different aspects of neck pain are covered including mechanics of collision impact and their rating, autopsy studies, dizziness and imbalance related to whiplash, and psychological aspects. The information assists in management of this widespread condition which is difficult to treat and requires a multimodality approach. The attempt to quantify disability and the review of physical, therapeutic and manipulative treatment techniques are notable. Several well known researchers contributed to this valuable book."

Andrew A. Fischer, MD, PhD
Associate Clinical Professor
of Rehabilitation Medicine
Mount Sinai School of Medicine (CUNY)
Chief, Physical Medicine
& Rehabilitation Service
VA Medical Center, Bronx, NY 10468

"In several of the chapters of this informative multi-authored book for the Banff Symposium on whiplash, the unresolved issue of causal relationship between chronic symptoms and injuries with whiplash mechanism is sensibly avoided. Patients complaints are instead taken at face value, an acceptable approach as long as one is aiming at better diagnosis and treatment and not at the support of financial claims.

In the first four chapters the authors address the problem of determining minimal impact severity that causes acute symptoms, and the role of accident mechanisms. Two articles review the scientific evidence on effectiveness of passive physical therapy, manipulation and mobilisation. Four chapters are devoted to psychological aspects of chronic pain as well as to treatment and coping strategies. In one section a newly developed neck disability index is presented. Other contributions are an autopsy study, investigations of cervical synovial joints and case studies of patients with dizziness and imbalance.

The majority of chapters are well written and readable. Special attention has to be drawn to the editorial by Allen and to the editorial on the Quebec Task Force on WAD by Cassidy as they offer excellent and critical views; worthwhile reading to anyone interested in this important and controversial public issue. The opinions expressed elsewhere in the book are also reasonably balanced. . . . Examples of chapters which could be singled out as particularly informative to the reader are the first two on minimal impact severity. These reviews are highly useful for medicolegal purposes. . . . Especially valuable for the treating physician are the chapters that empasize the need for individually-matched behavioral and cognitive coping strategies for pain and the necessity of therapy modalities that prevent evolution of chronicity."

Harald Schrader, MD, PhD
Professor of Clinical Neurology
Norwegian University of Science
and Technology
and Chief Physician at the Department
of Neurology, University Hospital of
Trondheim

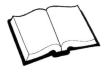

Musculoskeletal Pain Emanating from the Head and Neck

Current Concepts in Diagnosis, Management and Cost Containment

Musculoskeletal Pain Emanating from the Head and Neck

Current Concepts in Diagnosis, Management and Cost Containment

Murray E. Allen, MD
Editor

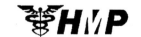

The Haworth Medical Press
An Imprint of
The Haworth Press, Inc.,
New York • London

Published by

The Haworth Medical Press, 10 Alice Street, Binghamton, NY 13904-1580 USA

The Haworth Medical Press is an imprint of the Haworth Press, Inc., 10 Alice Street, Binghamton, NY 13904-1580 USA.

Musculoskeletal Pain Emanating from the Head and Neck: Current Concepts in Diagnosis, Management and Cost Containment has also been published as *Journal of Musculoskeletal Pain*, Volume 4, Number 4 1996.

Library of Congress Cataloging-in-Publication Data

Musculoskeletal pain emanating from the head and neck : current concepts in diagnosis, management and cost containment / Murray E. Allen, editor.
     p. cm.–(Journal of musculoskeletal pain; v. 4, no. 4)
     Proceedings of the International Symposium on "Musculoskeletal Pain Emanating from the Head and Neck", held in Banff, Canada, Oct. 13-15, 1995.
     Includes bibliographical references and index.
     ISBN 0-7890-0005-9 (alk. paper)
     1. Neck pain–Congresses. 2. Headache–Congresses. 3. Whiplash injuries–Congresses. I. Allen, Murray. II. International Symposium on "Musculoskeletal Pain Emanating from the Head and Neck" (1995 : Banff, Alta.) III. Series.
     [DNLM: 1. Cervical Vertebrae–injuries–congresses. 2. Whiplash Injuries–complications–congresses. 3. Head Injuries–complications–congresses. 4. Pain–etiology–congresses. 5. Accidents, Traffic–congresses. W1 J0775RK v.4 no.4 1996 / WE 725 M985 1996]
RC936.M87 1996
617.5' 1–dc20
DNLM/DLC
for Library of Congress

96-31753
CIP

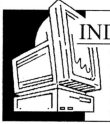

INDEXING & ABSTRACTING

Contributions to this publication are selectively indexed or abstracted in print, electronic, online, or CD-ROM version[s] of the reference tools and information services listed below. This list is current as of the copyright date of this publication. See the end of this section for additional notes.

- *Behavioral Medicine Abstracts,* Pain Evaluation and Treatment Institute, 4601 Baum Boulevard, Pittsburgh, PA 15213-1217

- *Behavioral Medicine Abstracts,* University of Washington, School of Social Work, Seattle, WA 98195

- *Cambridge Scientific Abstracts,* Environmental Routenet (accessed via INTERNET), 7200 Wisconsin Avenue #601, Bethesda, MD 20814

- *CFIDS Pathfinder,* P.O. Box 2644, Kensington, MD 20891-2644

- *CINAHL [Cumulative Index to Nursing & Allied Health Literature], in print, also on CD-ROM from CD PLUS, EBSCO, and SilverPlatter, and online from CDP Online [formerly BRS], Data-Star, and PaperChase. [Support materials include Subject Heading List, Database Search Guide, and instructional video],* CINAHL Information Systems, P.O. Box 871/1509 Wilson Terrace, Glendale, CA 91209-0871

- *CNPIEC Reference Guide: Chinese National Directory of Foreign Periodicals,* P.O. Box 88, Beijing, People's Republic of China

- *Dental Abstracts,* Mosby-Year Book, Inc., 200 N. LaSalle Street, Chicago, IL 60601-1080

- *Ergonomics Abstracts,* Taylor & Francis, Ltd., Rankine Road, Basingstoke, Hants RG24 0PR, England

- *Excerpta Medica/Secondary Publishing Division,* Elsevier Science Inc., Secondary Publishing Division, 655 Avenue of the Americas, New York, NY 10010

[continued]

- *Industrial Hygiene Digest,* Industrial Health Foundation, 34 Penn Circle West, Pittsburgh, PA 15206

- *Institute for Scientific Information,* 3501 Market Street, Philadelphia, Pennsylvania 19104. Coverage in:
  a) Social Science Citation Index [SSCI]: print, online, CD-ROM
  b) Research Alerts [current awareness service]
  c) Social SciSearch [magnetic tape]
  d) Current Contents/Social & Behavioral Sciencies [weekly current awareness service]

- *INTERNET ACCESS [& additional networks] Bulletin Board for Libraries ["BUBL"], coverage of information resources on INTERNET, JANET, and other networks.*
  - JANET X.29: UK.AC.BATH.BUBL or 00006012101300
  - TELNET: BUBL.BATH.AC.UK or 138.38.32.45 login 'bubl'
  - Gopher: BUBL.BATH.AC.UK [138.32.32.45]. Port 7070
  - World Wide Web: http://www.bubl.bath.ac.uk./BUBL/home.html
  - NISSWAIS: telnetniss.ac.uk [for the NISS gateway]
  The Andersonian Library, Curran Building, 101 St. James Road, Glasgow G4 ONS, Scotland

- *LifeSciences* .... see: *Institute for Scientific Information, Current Contents*

- *Pharmacist's Letter "Abstracts Section,"* Therapeutic Research Center, 8834 Hildreth Lane, Stockton, CA 95212

- *Physical Therapy "Abstracts Section,"* American Physical Therapy Association, 1111 North Fairfax Street, Alexandria, VA 22314-1488

- *Referativnyi Zhurnal [Abstracts Journal of the Institute of Scientific Information of the Republic of Russia],* The Institute of Scientific Information, Baltijskaja ul., 14, Moscow A-219, Republic of Russia

- *Sapient Health Network,* 10 NW 10th Avenue, Suite 430, Portland, OR 97209

- *Sport Database/Discus,* Sport Information Resource Center, 1600 James Naismith Drive, Suite 107, Gloucester, Ontario K1B 5N4, Canada

[continued]

SPECIAL BIBLIOGRAPHIC NOTES

related to special Journal issues [separates]
and indexing/abstracting

- ☐ indexing/abstracting services in this list will also cover material in any "separate" that is co-published simultaneously with Haworth's special thematic journal issue or DocuSerial. Indexing/abstracting usually covers material at the article/chapter level.

- ☐ monographic co-editions are intended for either non-subscribers or libraries which intend to purchase a second copy for their circulating collections.

- ☐ monographic co-editions are reported to all jobbers/wholesalers/approval plans. The source journal is listed as the "series" to assist the prevention of duplicate purchasing in the same manner utilized for books-in-series.

- ☐ to facilitate user/access services all indexing/abstracting services are encouraged to utilize the co-indexing entry note indicated at the bottom of the first page of each article/chapter/contribution.

- ☐ this is intended to assist a library user of any reference tool [whether print, electronic, online, or CD-ROM] to locate the monographic version if the library has purchased this version but not a subscription to the source journal.

- ☐ individual articles/chapters in any Haworth publication are also available through the Haworth Document Delivery Services [HDDS].

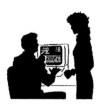

Musculoskeletal Pain Emanating from the Head and Neck

Current Concepts in Diagnosis, Management and Cost Containment

CONTENTS

ABOUT THE EDITOR

Murray Allen, MD, specializes in pain management and sports medicine at the medical consulting practice he established in North Vancouver, British Columbia. Prior to establishing private practice, Dr. Allen conducted musculoskeletal research as Associate Professor of Kinesiology at Simon Fraser University for 12 years. Dr. Allen is cofounder of the Metro Back Centre in Vancouver, and author of two popular books on exercise management of common neck and back problems. He is also a reviewer for granting agencies and scientific journals and has served as keynote speaker at many national and international scientific meetings.

Preface:
Musculoskeletal Pain Emanating from the Head and Neck:
A Proceedings Issue

The editor of this collection is Murray E. Allen, MD, who also served as the Chairman of the 8th International Symposium on "Musculoskeletal Pain Emanating from the Head and Neck" held in Banff, Canada, October 13-15, 1995.

Dr. Allen is a former Associate Professor of Kinesiology at Simon Fraser University and is currently a consultant in Musculoskeletal Medicine. He graduated in medicine from the University of Alberta in 1964 and pursued orthopedic postgraduate education related to musculoskeletal disorders. Later, as a faculty member at Simon Fraser University, he taught sports medicine courses and consulted on musculoskeletal medicine with an emphasis on sports medicine issues.

A recurring theme in Dr. Allen's publications has related to the role of exercise in elevating endogenous endorphins to physiologically produce what he refers to as the "runners calm" (1-3). His isokinetic research disclosed that high velocity movements represent somatic stresses which contribute to back and neck disorders (4). Dr. Allen's whiplash research involving motor vehicle accident simulations demonstrated that some routine activities of daily living can cause perturbations to the head and neck similar in magnitude to those resulting from low velocity rear-end collision injuries (5). This work broke new ground on how we view injury

[Haworth co-indexing entry note]: "Preface: Musculoskeletal Pain Emanating from the Head and Neck: A Proceedings Issue." Russell, I. Jon. Co-published simultaneously in *Journal of Musculoskeletal Pain* [The Haworth Medical Press, an imprint of The Haworth Press, Inc.] Vol. 4, No. 4, 1996, pp. xv-xvi and: *Musculoskeletal Pain Emanating from the Head and Neck: Current Concepts in Diagnosis, Management and Cost Containment* [ed: Murray E. Allen] The Haworth Medical Press, an imprint of The Haworth Press, Inc., 1996, pp. xiii-xiv. Single or multiple copies of this article are available from The Haworth Document Delivery Service [1-800-342-9678, 9:00 a.m. - 5:00 p.m. [EST]. E-mail address: getinfo@haworth.com].

xiii

dynamics. Finally, Dr. Allen has contributed to patient education with co-authored exercise books "Take Charge of Your Neck" and "Take Charge of Your Back" which teach isodynamic exercise (6).

I. Jon Russell, MD, PhD

REFERENCES

1. Allen ME, Thierman J, Hamilton D: Naloxone reverses the miosis in runners: Implications for an endogenous opiate test. Can J Appl Spt Sci 8: 98-103, 1983.

2. Allen ME, Coen D: Naloxone blocking of running-induced mood changes. Ann Sports Medicine 3: 190-195, 1987.

3. Allen ME: Endorphin: A role in sports medicine. Ann Sports Med 6: 23-31, 1991.

4. Allen ME: "Focus on Sportsmedicine" Clinical kinesiology: Measurement techniques for spinal disorders. Orthopaedic Rev 17: 1097-1104, 1988.

5. Allen ME, Weir-Jones I, Motiuk DR, Flewin KR, Goring RD, Kobetitch R, Broadhurst A: Acceleration perturbations of daily living, A comparison to "Whiplash." Spine 19: 1285-1290, 1994.

6. "Take Charge of Your Neck" and "Take Charge of Your Back" both published by Allen/Pothier, 1991.

EDITORIALS

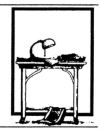

The New Whiplash

There are two great puzzles in this world that foster debate among humans, one is the wonder of the universe, the other is whiplash. For the first, Jupiter will soon be investigated by *Galileo*, the other [*whiplash*] was put into a new perspective at the 8th International Symposium by the Physical Medicine Research Foundation at Banff. What happens when the brightest minds on whiplash come together, do they consense?

The Quebec Task Force [QTF] (Cassidy) spent $3.5 million to determine a new name for whiplash, "*Whiplash Associated Disorder* [*WAD*]" and that for the most part we don't know what it is, nor what to do about it. In the first instance, we have failed to look at accident dynamics, and have made a vague assumption that all that collides will produce serious injury. Then our diagnostic acumen has been quite crude–we really don't know

[Haworth co-indexing entry note]: "The New Whiplash." Allen, Murray E. Co-published simultaneously in *Journal of Musculoskeletal Pain* [The Haworth Medical Press, an imprint of The Haworth Press, Inc.] Vol. 4, No. 4, 1996, pp. 1-4; and: *Musculoskeletal Pain Emanating from the Head and Neck: Current Concepts in Diagnosis, Management and Cost Containment* [ed: Murray E. Allen] The Haworth Medical Press, an imprint of The Haworth Press, Inc., 1996, pp. 1-4. Single or multiple copies of this article are available from The Haworth Document Delivery Service [1-800-342-9678, 9:00 a.m. - 5:00 p.m. [EST]. E-mail address: getinfo@haworth.com].

what goes wrong when it does go wrong. Also our sojourn over the last 20 years, wandering in the wilderness in search of a quick fix has not been fruitful. Have we manipulated our patients into a passive role, or lulled them with the expectation that some electric gizmo will do it for them? Can we snap or pop them into health? The answer is no! Neither can we simply talk them out of suffering. And it gets worse when the lawyers and courts attempt to play the role of the health professional by tempting whiplash with money. Overall, we're doing quite poorly on whiplash, but will probably do better with Galileo's observations on Jupiter. But not to be disheartened, new directions are being forged. The Banff Symposium (authors in parenthesis) came up with some valuable consensus.

The engineer reconstructionists (Gough, Bailey) have provided a new wrinkle and new terms to accompany whiplash. Bump studies with human volunteers have provided some very exciting information, and the Swedes (Ake Nygren) are looking at seat-backs and head-restraints that might provide better protection from rear-enders in the future. Generally, the harder we're hit, the harder we hurt. We all agree that injury is probable in the high velocity impacts, but at the low magnitude events, probably under 8 km/h change of velocity [ΔV] the injury exposure may be minimal, perhaps in the same realm as being disturbed by some routine events of daily living. If this is so, how does the health professional recognize a minimalist event? Fine tuning impact magnitude will probably remain as an engineering feat, but for the rest of us, the collision that shows "no damage" to bumpers probably falls into an event which should not expose a person to significant injury. Occupants of such minor collisions may sustain "whiplash type I" problems, but this is minor, and they should be reassured to continue at work, and keep up the momentum of their lives (Cassidy). Personal individual differences might increase injury exposure, and this now becomes the realm of the clinician (Croft).

Once injured, what comes next? Those hit hard take longer to recover, and have more physical and psychological problems as a result (Radanov). However, 75% of persons with significant injury still recover in about three months, and well over 90% by the first year regardless of age or sex (Cassidy). An interesting Japanese study (Naito) presented at the Symposium showed population outcomes among Tokyo whiplash patients that were almost exactly comparable to those seen in Quebec (Cassidy) and Switzerland (Radanov).

Most soft tissue sprains in the body heal, but what goes wrong with those that do not seem to recover, or do so slowly? The very serious neck injuries have shown very subtle tearing to the end plates of discs, and to facet joints (Taylor). These tissues heal slowly. Maybe if we inject these facet joints that will cure whiplash? Indeed, in some cases this appears to provide very impressive short term relief (Lord), but only provides diagnostic information without lasting benefit. Is this another effort on our part to find a quick fix; will it fail again?

There have been many perplexing symptoms associated with whiplash, some of which were thought to be quite sinister. Dizziness and imbalance was thought to come from damage to the inner ear (Mallinson). One series of posters at the Symposium (Karlberg) noted that treatment of the dizzy patient to improve neck motion also improved the dizziness. Radiating symptoms to arms and shoulders were once thought to be injury to these soft tissues, or nerve entrapment. But simple irritation of almost any neck tissue will give vague non-radicular pain into the shoulders and arms. The severity of the radiations need not follow the severity of the neck injury. We used to use collars, a la. the principles of "Hugh the rester" [Hugh Owen Thomas], but collars are probably contra-indicated for whiplash. They irritate jaws, foster joint adhesions, and lead to tissue atrophy. Patients become quite frightened by all the weird secondary symptoms associated with whiplash and with harmful treatments, and sometimes their fears can spiral them into serious dysfunction. We need to be alert to the many secondary manifestations of whiplash, test for the perception of dysfunction (Vernon), and be reassuring where possible. Most of all we must foster an atmosphere of confidence, reassurance, encourage very early activation, and help persons maintain the momentum of their lives (Bélanger).

When whiplash occurs, what do we do for it? *The New York Times* (1 May 1995) boldly commented on whiplash treatments as researched by Quebec Task Force, "Most don't work, and some may even be harmful." Physicians can be blamed for prescribing too many drugs, such as tranquilizers, muscle relaxants, and pain pills, most of which are probably an ugly approach to whiplash (Gillies). Physiotherapists are chided for excessive passive modalities which not only do no good, but by their repeated failure can help convince the poor suffering patients that all is lost. Failure to help is a contributor to harm (Bélanger). Among the chiropractors, repeated manipulations can also foster illness behavior, but short term manipulation and mobilization may be helpful (Vernon, Coulter).

As always, the last word goes to the mind-benders. Some acerbic cynics would foster the idea that chronic pain is all in the mind. Certainly the brain is the final arbiter of all that it perceives, and has been shown that with "focus on pain," one can enhance the suffering (Patrick Wall). But for those so suffering, the pain is very real, the anguish is truly felt. Are such chronic sufferers causing this to themselves, or did the whiplash lead them into it? Recent studies could not find any predisposing psychological profile that would predict chronic outcomes from injury (Radanov, Turk). Indeed, one small study found if the pain in a facet joint could be blocked, the depression would also resolve (Lord). Yet in chronic jaw joint complaints, the major associated factors were the psycho-social dysfunction, not the physical pathology (Dworkin). In other studies, there is a close link between physical suffering and psychosocial dysfunction, but which comes first has not been clearly solved (Marbach). Certainly treatments for chronic pain that do not take account of a person's psychosocial stress are probably doomed to failure (Main).

So where is new-whiplash leading us? Actually, we're going back to our roots, when whiplash was not a word, and its suffering was not a secondary benefit. First of all, as a primary premise, we must realize that, "all that whips is not lashed"; low velocity bumps do not dissolve someone's cervical spine. Remember the time when a "kink" in the neck meant you had to "work it out"? We call it "early activation" now, but it is still the same principle. We must boost our patients back into the main-stream of life, for if they lose their momentum, they may not get started again. Patience is a virtue; all sprains take months to heal, so don't be hasty in expecting instant quick fixes. We must stop most if not all drugs, avoid passive failure-mode treatments, and avoid prolonged medicalization of any form of treatment—we must foster self-reliance. Does this mean the stiff upper lip, the stoic? Probably yes! This means defocusing off pain, ignoring it, and getting on with life. But this has to be administered with a caring soft sell, not a rejection-mode turn-off. When all else fails and chronic pain dysfunction ensues, then the multi-disciplinary team is probably needed.

Will whiplash always be with us? As long as humans have large heads perched on top of flimsy spines, yes! But automobiles may not always be the cause. In a recent survey, one out-back doctor in Canada stated that the commonest cause of whiplash among his patients was from river rafting.

Murray E. Allen, MD

The Quebec Task Force
on Whiplash-Associated Disorders:
Implications for Clinical Management
and Future Directions for Research

J. David Cassidy

SUMMARY. With the recent publication of the *Scientific Monograph of the Quebec Task Force on Whiplash-Associated Disorders*, a baseline of clinical and scientific information was established. However, of the substantial number of publications reviewed by the Task Force, only a few met a priori scientific criteria for admissibility. This lack of scientific evidence placed some important limitations on the ability of the Task Force to recommend preventive, diagnostic and therapeutic measures for the management of whiplash and its associated disorders. In order to advance knowledge on this major public health problem, there will have to be a substantial improvement in the quality of published research. *[Article copies available from The Haworth Document Delivery Service: 1-800-342-9678. E-mail address: getinfo@haworth.com]*

J. David Cassidy, DC, PhD, FCCSC, is Research Director, Neuromusculoskeletal Health Center, University of Saskatchewan, Saskatoon, and Co-Author of the Quebec Task Force on Whiplash Associated Disorders.

Address correspondence to: J. David Cassidy, Centre for Neuromusculoskeletal Health, P.O. Box 108, Department of Orthopaedics, Royal University Hospital, 103 Hospital Drive, Saskatoon, Canada S7N 0W8.

[Haworth co-indexing entry note]: "The Quebec Task Force on Whiplash-Associated Disorders: Implications for Clinical Management and Future Directions for Research." Cassidy, J. David. Co-published simultaneously in *Journal of Musculoskeletal Pain* [The Haworth Medical Press, an imprint of The Haworth Press, Inc.] Vol. 4, No. 4, 1996, pp. 5-9; and: *Musculoskeletal Pain Emanating from the Head and Neck: Current Concepts in Diagnosis, Management and Cost Containment* [ed: Murray E. Allen] The Haworth Medical Press, an imprint of The Haworth Press, Inc., 1996, pp. 5-9. Single or multiple copies of this article are available from The Haworth Document Delivery Service [1-800-342-9678, 9:00 a.m. - 5:00 p.m. [EST]. E-mail address: getinfo@haworth.com].

KEYWORDS. Whiplash, task force, management

Recent figures show that the whiplash problem is substantial and growing. In the Canadian province of Quebec, approximately 5,000 whiplash injuries account for 20% of all compensated traffic injury claims annually. The average period for compensation for these injuries increased from 72 days in 1987 to 108 days in 1989 (1,2). In two other Canadian provinces with single-payer motor vehicle insurance programs, 68% of British Columbian claims and 85% of Saskatchewan claims were for whiplash injuries (2,3). Moreover, the incidence of whiplash injury varies greatly between different locations. In Quebec, the 1987 incidence of compensated whiplash claims was 70/100,000 inhabitants. In 1987 the Saskatchewan incidence of compensated whiplash claims was in excess of 700/100,000 inhabitants, more than a ten fold increase over Quebec. During that year, Quebec's insurance system was "no fault" [benefits are available regardless of fault for the collision, but claimants cannot sue for pain and suffering in excess of these benefits] while under the tort system in Saskatchewan, victims of collisions could sue for pain and suffering in excess of benefits. The implication of this finding is uncertain and could be partially explained by the way claims are counted. However, a cynical point of view would include the suggestion of monetary factors motivating whiplash claims (4). Recently, both Saskatchewan [1995] and Manitoba [1994] have changed to a no fault provincial insurance system that includes increased rehabilitation benefits. The impact of this change is currently being investigated in Saskatchewan.

Whiplash is to the automobile what low-back pain is to the workplace. However, unlike occupational low-back injuries, whiplash has not been subjected to such intense scientific study. For example, although there has been a great deal of research showing the importance of psychosocial factors in occupational low back pain, little has been published concerning these factors in neck pain after traffic injury. The notable exception to this is the work of Radanov and colleagues (5-8). This lack of attention is surprising considering the prevalence and burden of illness associated with neck pain after traffic collisions. During the first six months of 1992, Saskatchewan Government Insurance settled 2,658 whiplash claims at a cost of over $26,000,000 (3).

With the recent publication of the *Scientific Monograph of the Quebec Task Force on Whiplash-Associated Disorders*, a baseline of clinical and scientific information was established (9). Over the course of four years, a team of international scientists and clinicians applied the method of "best evidence synthesis" to the whiplash literature (10). They screened over

10,000 papers and abstracts identified in the English and French literature from September 1980 to September 1994. Of these, 1,204 were subjected to a preliminary review. Only 294 publications contained scientific data about whiplash. The 294 papers were then subjected to an in-depth review applying a priori rules for scientific admissibility. The Quebec Task Force [QTF] finally judged that only 62 papers were both scientifically acceptable and clinically relevant. These accepted studies formed the basis for the recommendations on diagnosis, prognosis, treatment and risk associated with whiplash.

Although there is a vast literature on the subject of whiplash, it is obviously of poor scientific quality. The QTF was not able to find one acceptable population-based study on the risk of whiplash associated disorder [WAD]. Although some authors published estimates of the problem, the population at risk was missing as a denominator. There were no acceptable studies documenting sensitivity, specificity and predictive values for diagnostic tests. Prognostic studies were generally small and lacking statistical power. Biased selection of study subjects was a major problem in most studies. The few randomized controlled trials of interventions in the literature were methodically weak, mixed treatment effects and were difficult to interpret.

The QTF recommended a simple classification system for differentiating mild, moderate and severe cases of WAD. A time-driven treatment algorithm based on expected healing times for soft-tissues and modified by the classification of the patient was proposed. The QTF published "Minimum Data Collection Forms" for clinicians, in the hope that the systematic collection of standardized clinical data would result in better criteria for prognosis and future research possibilities to validate the clinical classification. A subgroup of the QTF analyzed a retrospective cohort of 3,014 whiplash claims from the 1987 Quebec insurance data base. This showed that the vast majority of WAD victims recovered quickly, but that 12.5% of claimants still compensated six months after the collision accounted for 46% of the total cost to the insurance system.

The obvious lack of credible scientific data on whiplash underscores three important points:

1. Clinical approaches to the diagnosis and prognosis of whiplash need to be validated.
2. Most treatment and rehabilitation programs for persons with WAD have not been tested for their effectiveness.
3. Clinicians and research scientists need to collaborate more closely to advance the current state of knowledge through properly conducted scientific studies.

The first step toward a resolution to the problem of WAD is its recognition as an important public issue. The publication of the *Scientific Monograph of the Quebec Task Force on Whiplash-Associated Disorders* and other high profile reviews of the subject have focused attention on WAD (11,12). Major international conferences on this subject have been held recently in Stockholm and Banff (13,14). Insurance companies in Sweden and Canada are now funding scientific research into WAD. Scientists and clinicians spanning several disciplines are beginning to collaborate in treatment and research efforts. Political, economic and public pressure for effective and cost-effective management of WAD is growing. A new era of evidence-based medicine is coming. The next task force is to address the problem of WAD will hopefully find a more credible body of scientific knowledge on which to guide their recommendations.

AUTHOR NOTE

The consensus conference of experts at Banff (14) endorsed the findings and recommendations of the QTF, including the widespread use of the "Minimum Data Collection Forms."

REFERENCES

1. Girard N: Statisques descriptives sur la nature des blessures. Quebec: Régie de l'assurance automobile du Québec, Direction des services médicaux et de la réadaptation. Internal Document, 1989 avr.

2. Giroux M: Les blessures _ a la colonne cervicale: importance du probléme. le Médecin du Québec Sept 22-6, 1991.

3. Sobeco, Ernst and Young: Saskatchewan Government Insurance automobile injury study. Report to the Saskatchewan Government Insurance Office, March 1989.

4. Gotten N: Survey of one hundred cases of whiplash injury after settlement of litigation. JAMA 162: 865-867, 1956.

5. Radanov BP, Di Stefano G, Schnidrig A, Ballinari P: Role of psychosocial stress in recovery from common whiplash. Lancet 338: 712-5, 1991.

6. Radanov BP, Hirlinger I, Di Stefano G, Valach L: Attentional processing in cervical spine syndromes. Acta Neurol Scand 85: 358-62, 1992.

7. Radanov BP, Sturzenegger M, De Stefano G, Schnidrig A: Relationship between early somatic, radiological, cognitive and psychosocial findings and outcome during one-year follow-up in 117 patients suffering from common whiplash. Br J Rheumatol 33: 442-8, 1994.

8. Radanov BP, Sturzenegger M, Di Stefano G, Schnidrig A, Aljinovic M: Factors influencing recovery from headache after common whiplash. BMJ 307: 652-5, 1993.

9. Spitzer WO, Skovro ML, Salmi LR, Cassidy JD, Duranceau J, Suissa S, Zeiss E: Scientific monograph of the Quebec task force on whiplash-associated disorders: redefining "whiplash" and its management. Spine 20 (Suppl): 1S-73S, 1995.

10. Slavin RE: Best evidence synthesis: an alternative to meta-analytic and traditional reviews. Educational Researchers 15: 5-11, 1986.

11. Barnsley L, Lord S, Bogduk N: Whiplash injury. Pain 58: 283-307, 1994.

12. Ekholm J, Harms-Ringdahl K, Nygren A: Back to work: neck-and-shoulder problems. On mechanisms, individual and societal consequences, rehabilitation and prevention. Scand J Rehabil Med (Suppl 32): 1-127, 1995.

13. Whiplash-associated disorders: redefining whiplash and its management. Karolinska Institute and Folksham Research. Stockholm, May 1995.

14. Musculoskeletal pain emanating from the head and neck: current concepts in diagnosis, management and cost containment. Physical Medicine Research Foundation. Banff, Oct. 1995.

ARTICLES

Human Occupant Dynamics
in Low-Speed Rear End Collisions:
An Engineering Perspective

Jonathan P. Gough

SUMMARY. Over the past 50 years an extensive body of literature has been published on the topic of whiplash injuries resulting from rear end collisions. The hypothesized injury mechanisms have been varied and conflicting, suggesting a misunderstanding of the human occupant dynamics which occur in such collisions. Much of this misunderstanding may result from the use of anthropomorphic dummies in staged collision tests. Without knowledge of the mechanisms by which injuries are sustained, automobile design will be lacking in appropriate safety features. Without an understanding of injury mecha-

---

Jonathan P. Gough, BSc, PEng, is Reconstruction Engineer, Baker Materials Engineering Ltd., Vancouver, BC.

Address correspondence to: Jonathan P. Gough, Baker Materials Engineering Ltd., 2221 Manitoba Street, Vancouver, BC, Canada, V5Y 3A3.

[Haworth co-indexing entry note]: "Human Occupant Dynamics in Low-Speed Rear End Collisions: An Engineering Perspective." Gough, Jonathan P. Co-published simultaneously in *Journal of Musculoskeletal Pain* [The Haworth Medical Press, an imprint of The Haworth Press, Inc.] Vol. 4, No. 4, 1996, pp. 11-19; and: *Musculoskeletal Pain Emanating from the Head and Neck: Current Concepts in Diagnosis, Management and Cost Containment* [ed: Murray E. Allen] The Haworth Medical Press, an imprint of The Haworth Press, Inc., 1996, pp. 11-19. Single or multiple copies of this article are available from The Haworth Document Delivery Service [1-800-342-9678, 9:00 a.m. - 5:00 p.m. [EST]. E-mail address: getinfo@haworth.com].

11

nisms, health professionals may make incorrect assumptions about trauma severity and may render inappropriate treatment for sufferers. *[Article copies available from The Haworth Document Delivery Service: 1-800-342-9678. E-mail address: getinfo@haworth.com]*

KEYWORDS. Whiplash, occupant dynamics, motor vehicle accidents

INTRODUCTION

The term whiplash was coined in the mid 1940's to describe acute injury to the cervical spine resulting from motor vehicle accidents (1). Whiplash described the motion, and therefore an assumed mechanism of injury to the head/neck complex, rather than the injury itself. The term fell into common usage and is still used to describe apparent soft tissue injuries of the neck resulting most commonly from rear end motor vehicle collisions. The early design of vehicles gave little consideration to protecting the occupants from trauma. Seats designed to control excessive movement of the head and neck in rear end collisions were virtually unknown. In the past 50 years, the introduction of lap and shoulder seat belts, air bags, crumple zones, energy absorbing interior surfaces, and head restraints have all contributed to the reduction of injuries in motor vehicle collisions. However, complaints of soft tissue neck injuries in low-speed rear end collisions remain a significant problem.

HUMAN SUBJECTS vs. ANTHROPOMORPHIC DUMMIES

The earliest study of occupant dynamics in low-speed rear impacts was published by Severy et al. (2). This study of five staged rear-end collisions resulted in speed changes to the struck vehicle of 8.4 and 8.8 km/h with human subjects. The other three tests, resulting in speed changes of 5.7, 9.5 and 16.2 km/h, involved anthropomorphic dummies. Comparison of the head acceleration curves for the human and dummy at similar impact severities revealed significant differences in the induced response. The dummy response curves tended to have higher and more abrupt peaks than the human response curves. This lack of biofidelity of the anthropomorphic dummy neck has continued to plague research into the possible mechanisms of injury resulting from low-speed rear impacts (3,4). Even the newer Hybrid III test dummy lacks sensitivity to the ΔV [change of velocity] both in angular excursion and rotational accelerations, and appears to be a poor human surrogate for predicting whiplash injury (3). In the field of human testing, utmost caution is the order to prevent injury to human test subjects, usually by conducting impacts at velocities below presumed injury thresholds.

EARLY INVESTIGATIONS OF WHIPLASH MECHANICS

The early studies by Severy (2) noted that forces acting on the struck vehicle caused it to be accelerated to its maximum speed within approximately 200 milliseconds. Movement of the test subject's head did not begin until the acceleration of the vehicle was almost complete. However, the subject's torso, which was in integral contact with the seat back, began its forward movement shortly after the initial contact between the vehicles. In a rear-end "whiplash" event, the mass of the head atop a flexible neck allows the head to be whipped first rearward and then forward relative to the torso. Injuries were postulated to occur either as a consequence of hyperextension and/or hyperflexion of the neck.

In 1967, Mertz and Patrick (5) tested a human [only one], cadavers, and anthropomorphic dummies in order to establish an injury mechanism in low-speed rear impacts. An acceleration/deceleration sled was utilized for the impact tests, which assessed impact severity, seat back rigidity, and head restraints effectiveness. However, the response of the sled's seat back under impact conditions would not have necessarily simulated the response of an automobile seat, nor of a real world vehicle-to-vehicle collision. The dynamics experienced by the two anthropomorphic dummies used by Mertz and Patrick were observed to correspond poorly with each other, with the cadaver test subjects, and with the single human test subject. The cadavers were observed to have similar response characteristics to each other, although again their motion corresponded poorly with that of the human subject. They did note that head-restraints were effective in reducing injury exposure, and that higher head accelerations were produced when the head was farther from the head-restraint. They concluded that the critical factor in the causation of neck injury in low-speed rear impacts was cervical torque rather than shear or axial forces acting on the cervical spine. Work of this nature lead to the introduction of mandatory head restraints in North American vehicles and has encouraged the use of properly adjusted head restraints.

A subsequent study (6) reported on the flexion and extension characteristics of the human cervical spine. They proposed a voluntary response envelope for torque, measured at the occipital condyles, as a function of angle of cervical extension. It was concluded that cervical torque, rather than angle of cervical extension was a better measure of injury exposure. They found that once the limits of the normal range of motion of the neck were reached, large increases in torque occurred for small increases in the angle of extension.

Despite the finding that properly adjusted head-restraints would prevent or reduce cervical hyperextension from occurring in low-speed rear impacts, whiplash injuries continued to be reported based on tests conducted with anthropomorphic dummies. A differential rebound theory proposed that the occupant's torso began to rebound from the seat back while the head was still moving rearward. This forward movement of the torso would then allow the neck to move into hyperextension, regardless of the height of the headrest. However, recent tests conducted using human test subjects have revealed that this differential rebound phenomenon does not occur.

RECENT INVESTIGATIONS OF WHIPLASH

Recent investigations have involved a variety of male and female subjects ranging in age from 22 to 63 years who experienced impact speed changes ranging from 2 to 16 km/h (3,7-14). These studies considered subjective evaluation of the test subjects along with high speed cinematography, videography, accelerometers, magnetic resonance imaging, cineradiography and electromyography [Table 1].

These studies have provided a good understanding of rear-end occupant dynamics, but still failed to answer the critical question on exact injury mechanism[s]. However, they revealed a possible threshold above which normal human test subjects may experience some minor transient whiplash associated symptoms. Although cervical hyperextension is a probable injury mechanism which may occur in higher severity impacts where adequate head support is not available, it does not appear to be the sole mechanism of injury. In impacts where the struck vehicle's speed change is less than 8 km/h, the range of cervical motion is generally confined within the subject's normal range, regardless of the degree of support afforded by the headrest. However, in all of the tests for speed changes up to and, in some cases, significantly in excess of 8 km/h, if symptoms were experienced, they were minor and resolved spontaneously within hours to days. A speed change of 8 km/h may be a threshold below which injury is not expected.

In a low-speed rear impact, the collision forces cause the struck vehicle to be rapidly accelerated, usually from a stopped position. Under the idealized conditions used for testing with impact sleds, the sled is acceler-

TABLE 1. Studies of Low-Speed Rear End Collisions Using Human Subjects.

Author	Test Subjects ΔV km/h*	Impact	Assessment
West (7)	4 males ages 25 to 43 years	2 to 16	Subjective, accelerometers, videography.
McConnell (8)	4 males ages 45 to 56 years	3.0 to 8.1	Subjective, accelerometers, high speed cinematography.
Siegmund (13)	males and females ages unknown	1.7 to 8.8	Subjective.
Szabo (9)	3 males, 28 to 48 yrs 2 females, 27 to 58 yrs	approx. 8	Subjective, accelerometers, pre-post-test MRI.**
Siegmund (14)	2 males, 25 and 32 years	5.8 to 7.7	Subjective, amusement bumper cars.
Ono (10)	3 males, 22 to 43 yrs	4 to 8	Subjective, impact sled, electromyography, accelerometers, videography.
Rosenbluth (11)	1 male, 63 yrs 1 female, 55 yrs	3.3 to 7.8	Subjective, accelerometers.
Matsushita (12)	15 males, 22 to 61 yrs 3 females, 24 to 57 yrs	2.5 to 5.0	Subjective, electromyography, accelerometers, high speed cinematography and cineradiography.
Scott (3)	1 male, 50 years	3.9 to 7.8	Subjective, accelerometers, high speed cinematography.

*ΔV change of velocity in kilometers per hour
**MRI, magnetic resonance imaging

ated entirely along the longitudinal axis. However, in vehicle-to-vehicle impacts, the contacting surfaces of the two vehicles are not always flat and perfectly aligned. This can give rise to additional accelerations in the vertical plane which may effect occupant dynamics.

Seats in current model passenger vehicles come in a variety of designs. Headrests may be integral to the seat back or separate; canted forward or aligned with the seat back; present or absent. Seat back angles may be varied over a wide range to suit the physical characteristics and personal preferences of the vehicle occupants. However, regardless of the specific vehicle/occupant combination, seat backs are always angled rearward with respect to the vertical plane. As the vehicle is accelerated forward by the collision forces, not only is the torso accelerated forward by the seat back but it is also accelerated, to a smaller degree, in a vertical direction as a consequence of the inclination of the seat back. This causes a "ramping" of the torso up the seat back which can give rise to transient compressive stresses in the cervical spine. These spinal tension-compression forces have been proposed as a possible injury mechanism (8) in low-speed rear impacts, although no comparison between the levels of these forces in rear end collisions and those resulting from other human activities has been made. Some researchers have reported the head accelerations measured during normal activities (4,11,15), however, without simultaneous measurement of the accelerations of the lower cervical spine it is not possible to calculate the precise tension-compression stresses which may act on the cervical spine during these activities.

An early straightening of the initial curvature of lumbar lordosis and thoracic kyphosis which occurs at the beginning of ramping, may also give rise to vertical movement to the cervical spine. The portion of the vertical movement occurring as a consequence of seat back inclination may be predicted from consideration of the angle of the seat back and the magnitude of the vehicle acceleration. However, the portion which occurs as a consequence of straightening of the lumbar and thoracic spine would vary between individuals, depending on the initial degree of spinal curvature. It would be premature to modify seat design parameters to control this axial movement until the hypothesis that the axial cycling of the cervical spine is an actual mechanism of injury is demonstrated to be valid.

A recent detailed impact sled study of occupant dynamics in rear end collisions using automobile seats tested speed changes of 2.5 to 5.0 km/h (12). Cervical cineradiography recorded 90 images per second at impact, and compared the motion parameters to normal end range of motion on flexion-extension radiographs. Four out of 26 subjects reported minor localized neck ache which was first noticed on the morning following testing and resolved spontaneously within two to four days. Comparison of the exposure of these four individuals with that of the other test subjects revealed no pattern. Measures of age, sex, initial posture, initial muscle tension, head acceleration, and cervical motion parameters were the same for the minor symptomatic group and the asymptomatic group. [One of the rear ended subjects was leaning forward at the time of impact and complained of lumbar pain following testing. This seated position is atypical of the normal rear impact scenario and has not been considered in the following discussion.] Still, this study did not find an injury mechanism. Also, the short duration of the symptoms was not consistent with the effects of significant soft tissue injury.

The cineradiography films did, however, reveal several patterns of occupant dynamics which depended on the position initially adopted by the test subjects. Individuals who were leaning forward experienced an initial extension of the thoracic spine which resulted in an upward movement of the base of the cervical spine. As the base of the cervical spine moved upward, the inertia of the head prevented a simultaneous upward movement of the upper cervical spine. This resulted in the cervical spine experiencing compressive stresses. However, there did not appear to be a relationship between the magnitude of this compressive stress and the subsequent appearance of symptoms. An interesting consequence of this upward movement of the base of the cervical spine was that the initial movement of the cervical spine was flexion rather than extension for the forward leaners.

Individuals who were initially seated in an upright or reclined posture experienced an initial extension movement of their cervical spines as their heads were displaced rearward relative to their torsos. The lower cervical spine did not experience any upward movement as a result of straightening of the thoracic curvature and therefore no compression forces were experienced by the cervical spine. The severity of the impacts experienced by these subjects was below the level at which torso ramping is observed. None of the test subjects experienced hyperextension or hyperflexion of their cervical spines. This confirms earlier studies which have indicated that short term symptoms in rear impacts may not be dependent on hyperextension of the cervical spine.

Several researchers (4,16-18) have attempted to assess the statistical frequency with which whiplash occurs. Most epidemiologic studies are seriously flawed by the sampling technique. Typically, the data base is obtained by consideration of police reports, individuals reporting to trauma centers, tow away accidents, or other such criteria. Subjective complaints of injury are accepted without question and the estimates of impact severity are often poorly conceived. Statistical studies of injury potential in rear end collisions [of usually unknown severity] are usually of little value. Other researchers (19,20) have reported that whiplash injuries are frequently exaggerated or falsified.

Research which has involved live human subjects has principally involved speed changes of less than 8 km/h, although some have gone up to 16 km/h. Without exception, these tests have resulted in the subjects experiencing no significant or lasting symptoms. In fact, in cases where symptoms were reported, these symptoms always resolved spontaneously, without treatment, within a short period of time. In contrast, rear impacts resulting in speed changes of only 2 to 3 km/h are often claimed to have resulted in disabling and sometimes widespread injuries. In the absence of some intervening factor which has a significant adverse effect on the susceptibility to injury of these individuals, such claims of injury cannot be rationalized with the available research into occupant dynamics in low-speed rear end collisions. Medical treatment of individuals who have experienced such minor collisions is often based on an assumption of hyperextension/hyperflexion injury to the cervical spine which as discussed above could not likely have occurred. Current research indicates that this mechanism of injury does not occur for impacts resulting in a speed change of less than 8 km/h.

CONCLUSIONS

Early studies of the whiplash phenomenon concluded that in rear end collisions, injury to the cervical spine was a direct consequence of hyperextension and/or hyperflexion of the neck. Seat designs of that era did not provide any support for the head and neck and thus, it was possible for hyperextension of the neck to occur. When hyperextension does occur, injury to the neck can be expected.

Current automobile seats have evolved significantly from those of the 1940's. When properly designed, they provide excellent support for the head and neck and will prevent cervical hyperextension from occurring. If the early whiplash models were correct, prevention of cervical hyperextension would be expected to prevent whiplash injuries from occurring. This does not appear to be the case. This indicates that while cervical hyperextension is one mechanism by which whiplash injuries can occur in rear impacts, it may not be the only mechanism.

Recent studies of human occupant dynamics in low-speed rear end collisions have revealed previously unknown components of the motion of the head and cervical spine. However, these studies have not revealed any clear mechanism by which injury to the cervical spine can occur. At best, we can state that cervical hyperextension may not be the sole mechanism of injury to the cervical spine in rear end collisions. Other injury mechanisms have been proposed but none of these have been confirmed by testing of human subjects.

In staged tests conducted using human volunteers, no significant symptoms have been reported for speed changes of less than 8 km/h. In contrast, impacts of this severity frequently result in claims of disabling injury by the general public. The reasons for this incongruity have not been, and may not be, explained by occupant dynamics.

REFERENCES

1. Davis AG: Injuries of the cervical spine. JAMA 127[3]: 149-156, 1945.

2. Severy DM, Mathewson JH, Bechtol CO: Controlled automobile rear-end collisions, an investigation of related engineering and medical phenomena. Canadian Services Medical J 11[10]: 727-759, 1955.

3. Scott MW, McConnell WE, Guzman HM, et al.: Comparison of human and ATD head kinematics during low-speed rearend impacts. SAE 930094: 1993.

4. States JD, Balcerak JC, Williams JS, et al.: Injury frequency and head restraint effectiveness in rear-end impact accidents. Proc of the Sixteenth Stapp Car Crash Conf: 228-255, 1972.

5. Mertz HJ, Patrick LM: Investigation of the kinematics and kinetics of whiplash. SAE 670919: 1967.

6. Mertz HJ, Patrick LM: Strength and response of the human neck. SAE 710855: 1971.

7. West DH, Gough JP, Harper GTK: Low speed rear-end collision testing using human subjects. Accident Reconstruction J 5[3]: 22-26, 1993.

8. McConnell WE, Howard RP, Guzman HM, et al.: Analysis of human test subject kinematic responses to low velocity rear end impacts. SAE 930889: 1993.

9. Szabo TJ, Welcher JB, Anderson RD, et al.: Human occupant kinematic response to low speed rear-end impacts. SAE 940532: 1994.

10. Ono K, Kanno M: Influences of the physical parameters on the risk to neck injuries in low impact speed rear-end collisions. Proc of the 1993 International IRCOBI Conf on the Biomechanics of Impacts: 201-212, 8-10 September 1993, Eindhoven, Netherlands.

11. Rosenbluth W, Hicks L: Evaluating low-speed rear-end impact severity and resultant occupant stress parameters. J of Forensic Sci 39[6]: 1393-1424, 1994.

12. Matsushita T, Sato TB, Hiraboyashi K, et al.: X-ray study of the human neck motion due to head inertia loading. SAE 942208: 1994.

13. Siegmund GP, Bailey MN, King DJ: Characteristics of specific automobile bumpers in low-velocity impacts. SAE 940916: 1994.

14. Siegmund GP, Williamson PB: Speed change [ΔV] of amusement park bumper cars. Proceedings of the Canadian Multidisciplinary Road Safety Conf VIII: 299-308, 14-16 June 1993.

15. Allen ME, Weir-Jones I, Motiuk DR, et al.: Acceleration perturbations of daily living, a comparison to "whiplash." Spine 19[11]: 1285-1290, 1994.

16. Otremski I, Marsh JL, Wilde BR, et al.: Soft tissue cervical spinal injuries in motor vehicle accidents. Injury: The British J of Accident Surgery 20[6]: 349-351, 1989.

17. Carlson WL: AID analysis of national accident summary. HIT Lab Reports: 1971.

18. Kihlberg JK: Flexion-torsion neck injury in rear impacts. Proc Thirteenth Annual Meeting AAAM: 1-16, 1969.

19. Bramstein PW, Moore JO: The fallacy of the term "whiplash injury." Am J of Surgery 97: 522-529, 1959.

20. Gotten N: Survey of one hundred cases of whiplash injury after settlement of litigation. JAMA 162: 865-867, 1959.

Assessment of Impact Severity in Minor Motor Vehicle Collisions

Mark Bailey

SUMMARY. Objectives. To categorize common types of minor collisions, relate vehicle motion from minor collisions to various descriptors of impact severity, and to review the relevance of impact severity to the potential for injury in different minor collision types.

Findings. Descriptors of impact severity for a vehicle in a collision include velocity change [ΔV], equivalent barrier speed [EBS], peak acceleration, and vibration dose value [VDV]. Impact severity in terms of ΔV and EBS can be deduced from vehicle damage. Based on responses of human volunteers who were present in staged-collision tests, correlations were made between the various descriptors of impact severity and human volunteer response. Minor, short duration symptoms occur in rear-end collisions at the 8 km/h ΔV level; symptoms are not observed in frontal or lateral collisions until about 2 to 3 times this level. In rear end collisions the 8 km/h ΔV level can sometimes be achieved without vehicle damage.

Conclusions. Impact severity appears to be an influential variable in minor automobile collisions. Responses of volunteers in minor collisions indicate that symptoms are non-existent in very minor im-

Mark Bailey, BASc, MASc, is Reconstruction Engineer, Macinnis Engineering Associates Ltd., Vancouver, BC.

Address correspondence to: Mark Bailey, Macinnis Engineering Associates Ltd., 11-11151 Horseshoe Way, Richmond, BC, Canada, V7A 4S5.

The author would like to acknowledge Michael Gardiner for a review of the human volunteer literature, Jonathan Lawrence and David Garau for collision testing.

[Haworth co-indexing entry note]: "Assessment of Impact Severity in Minor Motor Vechicle Collisions." Bailey, Mark. Co-published simultaneously in *Journal of Musculoskeletal Pain* [The Haworth Medical Press, an imprint of The Haworth Press, Inc.] Vol. 4, No. 4, 1996, pp. 21-38; and: *Musculoskeletal Pain Emanating from the Head and Neck: Current Concepts in Diagnosis, Management and Cost Containment* [ed: Murray E. Allen] The Haworth Medical Press, an imprint of The Haworth Press, Inc., 1996, pp. 21-38. Single or multiple copies of this article are available from The Haworth Document Delivery Service [1-800-342-9678, 9:00 a.m. - 5:00 p.m. [EST]. E-mail address: getinfo@haworth.com].

21

pacts, and worsen as severity is increased. Other variables are seat type, posture, gender, age and physical condition. *[Article copies available from The Haworth Document Delivery Service: 1-800-342-9678. E-mail address: getinfo@haworth.com]*

KEYWORDS. Collision, whiplash, injury, engineering, reconstruction

COLLISION RECONSTRUCTION

Four types of "minor" collisions frequently occur. These are rear-end, front-end, lateral, and side-swipe. The reconstructionist's term "minor" is used to describe impacts where tire forces and/or restitution effects cannot be ignored. It is not used to reference vehicle damage or occupant symptoms, though vehicles often display either no, or only minor damage. Objective clinical findings may be absent in the victim of a minor collision, so that all of the diagnosis is subjective. One objective finding that is often overlooked is the collision itself. The variables are the collision type and the collision severity. Minor collision severity can be quantified with some precision based on the post-collision condition of the vehicle[s]. Severity may predicate injury exposure.

Human tolerance data for the collision types is derived from staged collision tests where there were human volunteer occupants. Collision severity is compared to the subjective response which can range from no symptoms to minor symptoms which resolved in a few minutes to a few days.

In *rear-end [front-end] collisions*, the struck, or target, vehicle experiences a rear-end collision and the striking, or bullet, vehicle a front-end collision. The two vehicles may be offset or at a small angle. In passenger cars, the bumper heights are normally equal enough that the collision is bumper to bumper. If one vehicle has a high bumper [a truck for example] or if the striking vehicle's front bumper is pitched down from heavy braking, then the bumper heights will not match and one vehicle will go beneath the other. This is known as an under-ride or override engagement.

In *lateral collisions*, the front or back bumper of the bullet vehicle hits the side of the target vehicle. Damage is more extensive on the struck vehicle since the side body panels [struck vehicle] are weaker than bumpers [striking vehicle]. Lateral collisions also occur in lane changes when the two vehicles are moving at nearly equal speeds and the side of the striking vehicle moves sideways into the side of the struck vehicle.

Side-swipe collisions involve localized damage on one vehicle and a larger zone of damage on the other vehicle. A local area of the striking vehicle, such as the corner of the front bumper, scrapes past the side of the struck vehicle, creating creases, dents and sometimes snags.

Velocity change [Delta V, ΔV] can be applied to all types and severities of collisions; ΔV is the nearly instantaneous change in a vehicle's speed and direction that results from an impact. Figure 1 shows the concept of velocity change in a minor rear impact. The stationary front car [the target] is hit by the rear car moving at 10 km/h [the bullet]. After the vehicles

FIGURE 1. Velocity change in rear and front impacts. Both vehicles experience 7 km/h ΔV.

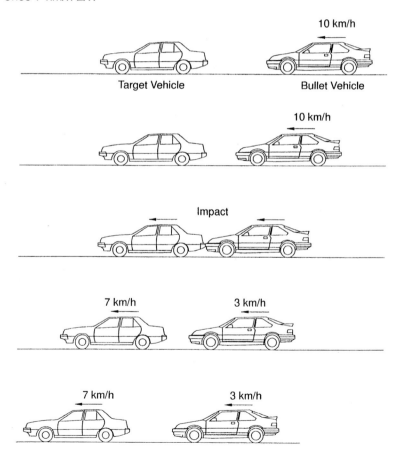

collide and separate, the target has a velocity of 7 km/h. Since its initial velocity was zero, its velocity change was 7 km/h [impact severity = 7 km/h ΔV]. Velocity change is a preferred descriptor of impact severity because it can be computed from vehicle damage after an impact, it is relevant to occupant motion, and it correlates to injury outcome.

Equivalent Barrier Speed [EBS] is a related concept as illustrated in Figure 2. The car moves backward toward the barrier at 5 km/h, its EBS, rebounds forward at 2 km/h resulting in a 7 km/h ΔV. For the same impact speed, different cars will rebound at different speeds because of different

FIGURE 2. Equivalent Barrier Speed [EBS]. The vehicle strikes the wall at 5 km/h [EBS = 5 km/h] then rebounds at 2 km/h. Its Velocity Change is 7 km/h.

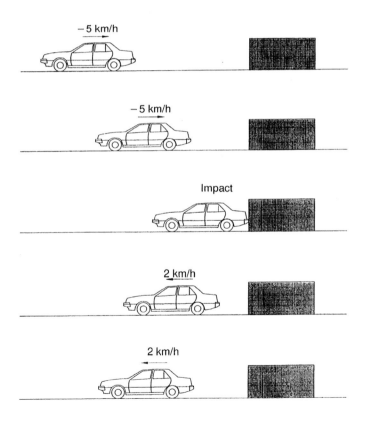

restitution [rebound factor of the bumper]. For front and rear impacts the rebound can be significant as shown in numerous staged collisions, and varies from about 0.3 to 0.7 of the EBS (1,2,3). A different rebound speed results in a different velocity change for the same EBS.

Acceleration is a measure of the rate of change of velocity. If the rate of change of velocity was steady, then the acceleration would be constant. However, this is not the case and there are complex acceleration peaks that are attributable to the involved vehicles. There are many identifiable acceleration peaks in the impact, but the highest of the peaks is usually termed the "vehicle peak acceleration" [Figure 3]. It generally occurs about half way through the impact, and hence will generally occur before significant occupant motion begins. However, different peak accelerations can occur for the same ΔV because of differences in impact duration [Figure 4].

Vibration dose value [VDV] has been used to help quantify vehicle ride, seat comfort and motion sickness. It uses the acceleration-time history of vehicle's motion to compute the VDV for that motion. It is applicable to vibratory motions which may be steady-state, random or transient. The VDV can be used to characterize the motion when there are occasional peaks above the background, termed high crest factor vibrations where crest factor is the ratio of peak to Root Mean Square acceleration (4). It has been suggested that a VDV of 15 ms$^{-1.75}$ is a level above which "some consideration of the health effects of the vibration may be appropriate." Figure 5 shows that a velocity change of 8 km/h in a rear end impact reaches the 15 ms$^{-1.75}$ level. Minor symptoms have occurred in human volunteers at that severity level. Use of the VDV is advantageous because it considers the effects of both peaks and background accelerations, as well as the duration of the disturbance. It may be applied to all types of minor impacts, but is most useful for side-swipes, which are characterized by long duration. It is not easily computed from vehicle damage, but can be easily computed from acceleration data from, for example, a vehicle equipped with a crash recorder, which may beocme a new trend.

Impact speed in itself is not a direct measure of impact severity. It can however be used to establish an approach speed which can then be used to compute ΔV if the vehicle masses and coefficient of restitution are known. The principle of conservation of momentum is also applied.

The *distance a vehicle moved* forward after an impact usually does not provide a reliable way to estimate closing speeds or speed changes. The distance a vehicle rolls forward after being hit depends on when and how hard the brakes were applied. Also, estimates of distance may be unreliable.

FIGURE 3. Acceleration trace for the vehicle in Figure 4. The "vehicle peak acceleration" is not the only peak in the trace, but is the highest trace.

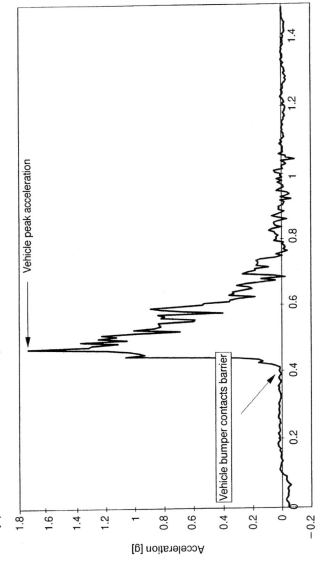

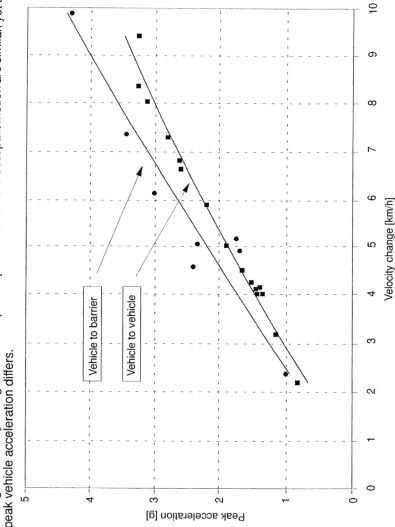

FIGURE 4. Comparison of peak vehicle acceleration and velocity change for vehicle to barrier and vehicle to vehicle impacts. Each data point represents one collision. There was no vehicle damage. For a given velocity change the vehicle post-impact condition and occupant motion are similar, yet the peak vehicle acceleration differs.

FIGURE 5. Comparison of Vibration Dose Value [VDV] and peak vehicle acceleration for vehicle to barrier impacts. A single impact is plotted as a single data point on each curve.

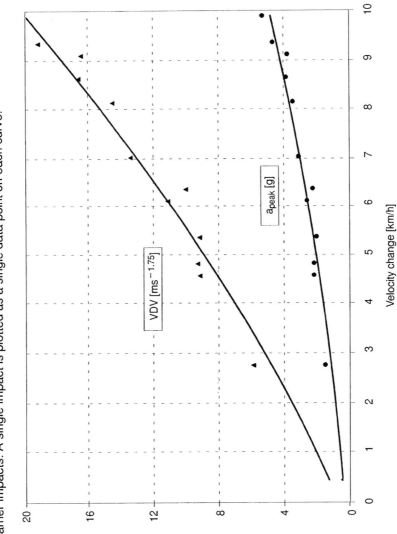

VEHICLE DAMAGE vs. IMPACT SEVERITY

In general terms, the severity of an impact is related to vehicle damage. A vehicle that has been crushed several centimeters on its rear has experienced a more severe impact than the same vehicle that has less or even no permanent rear-end damage. However, there are significant differences between the relative strengths of different surfaces of the same car, and between the same surfaces of different cars. For example, the rear ends of two different cars will not be equally strong, so that two different cars with similar damage may not have experienced the same impact severity.

Where there is bumper engagement with no damage in a rear or front impact, it is often possible to determine impact severity from an inspection of the vehicle bumpers. In many cases the amount of compression of a shock-absorber-like bumper component known as an isolator can be correlated to the vehicle's ΔV or EBS in a minor front or rear impact (2,5,6). In non-isolator equipped cars, which are increasingly more common, the task of determining severity is more difficult. For many passenger cars in North America, there is often little or no damage after a minor impact. Some Asian cars in particular have quite robust foam-core bumpers that are more damage resistant.

In lateral and side-swipe impacts the damage is more noticeable, since the body panels, which are much weaker than bumpers, are involved. Body panel dents and horizontal scuffs and creases are easily produced with very minor impacts.

Determining impact severity precisely requires a knowledge of some principles of physics, as well as damage properties or crush characteristics of the particular vehicles involved. The physical principles are conservation of momentum, conservation of energy, Newton's Third Law, and restitution (5).

Determining impact severity with much less precision only requires a knowledge of the type of impact and a general description of the vehicle damage. In a general sense, it is possible to apply Table 1, while emphasizing that each impact is different and exceptions exist. The "potential for symptoms" data come from staged collisions with optimally seated healthy young male volunteers. Symptoms may differ for accident victims not in this population group for reasons of age, health, gender, or posture. Symptoms may also differ for accident victims who do fall into this population group owing to differences in injury tolerance.

OCCUPANT MOTIONS

In any of the impact types, the initial occupant motion is generally toward the location where the collision force is applied. Hence in rear

TABLE 1. Comparison of Impact Type, Severity, and Symptoms in Healthy Male Volunteers in Typical Staged Collisions of Similar Severity.

Impact type	Damage	Impact km/h ΔV^*	Range of symptoms
rear	bumper engaged, no cosmetic, structural or other damage	16	insufficient data above 9 km/h ΔV
	bumper not engaged, none or very minor trunk or tail light damage	8	none, to neck/head/back ache/stiffness/discomfort lasting <24 h
front	bumper engaged, no cosmetic or structural damage; air-bag not deployed	16	none, to minor neck pain; "ouch" level
	minor damage to grille, headlights, bumper; no air-bag deployment	22	none, to neck pain, chest pain, back pain or headache
lateral	very minor body panel damage, no wheels or tires hit	8	none
side-swipe	very minor body panel damage, no snags, no wheels or tires hit	8	none, to neck/head/back ache/stiffness/discomfort lasting <24 h

*ΔV = velocity change

impacts, occupants move rearward relative to the vehicle, in front impacts they move toward the front and in lateral impacts, they move toward the struck side of the vehicle.

Staged vehicle impact tests with human volunteers have revealed that the velocity change of a vehicle in a minor collision is essentially complete before the occupant's head is displaced (7,8,9). Because the vehicle collision is mostly finished before the occupant's head moves, the velocity change is a measure of the speed at which the occupant head interferes with the vehicle interior, the so-called "human collision."

One retrospective study of automobile crashes (6) related severity to injury outcome using ΔV. It was found that there was a trend of increased AIS [Abbreviated Injury Scale] for increased velocity change in rear, front and lateral collisions ranging in severity from 16 to 100 km/h ΔV. In human volunteer testing it has also been found that symptoms worsen as ΔV is increased.

Impact studies have shown that even some of the most sophisticated anthropomorphic dummies have poor biofidelity regarding neck and head motions in minor rear impacts (7,8,10). This has lead researchers to use human volunteers in staged collisions that are at presumed sub-injury threshold collision severities. Overall, the motions of human volunteer occupants even at very low severities are too complex for simple correlation to exist between vehicle impact severity and single descriptors of occupant motion. For example, there does not appear to be a precise correlation between vehicle impact severity and head peak acceleration for different vehicles [Figure 6].

Szabo (8) showed in a series of 8 km/h ΔV rear end impacts that there was a consistent pattern of motion for nearly identical impacts [same vehicle and same severity] even though the male and female volunteers had different ages and statures. Two phases of the impact were identified: in Phase 1 which ended 110 to 170 ms after initial vehicle contact, the vehicle moved forward beneath the occupant, so that the occupant moved rearward relative to the vehicle. The velocity change was complete after approximately 100 ms. In some cases the driver's hands came off the steering wheel. Phase 2 lasted 150 to 230 ms, where the occupant's upper torso contacted the seat back and head restraint. All significant motions were confined to the sagittal plane. None of the volunteers experienced neck hyperextension, but some experienced transient headaches which occurred immediately after impact and resolved spontaneously.

Similar results were presented in a later study by McConnell et al. (9). It was found that minor symptoms, such as neck discomfort or neck ache lasting a few hours, were generated in the male test subjects, but that neck hyperextension did not occur. Impact severities in the rear end collisions ranged from 4 to 8 km/h ΔV in four different vehicles. The symptoms worsened as the severity increased.

In rare instances it is possible for a driver in a rear-ended car to receive minor facial injuries. A Transport Canada study (11) was initiated in response to complaints of seat belt restrained drivers who had made contact with the steering wheel as a result of forward rebound out of the seat back after a rear-end collision. It was hypothesized that the seat belt

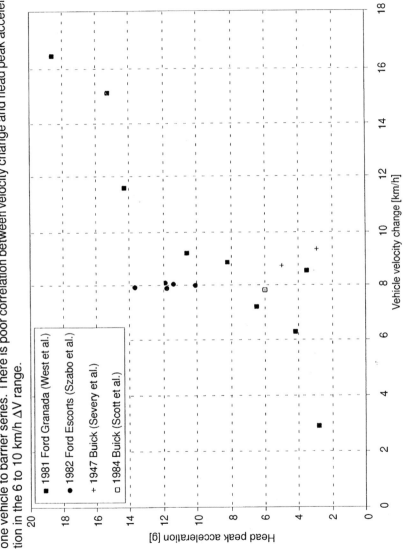

FIGURE 6. Comparison of vehicle velocity change and head peak acceleration for volunteers in staged minor rear-end vehicle to vehicle collisions. The data are from three different vehicle to vehicle pairs and one vehicle to barrier series. There is poor correlation between velocity change and head peak acceleration in the 6 to 10 km/h ΔV range.

- ■ 1981 Ford Granada (West et al.)
- ● 1982 Ford Escorts (Szabo et al.)
- + 1947 Buick (Severy et al.)
- □ 1984 Buick (Scott et al.)

Head peak acceleration [g]

Vehicle velocity change [km/h]

locking mechanism did not function in these rear impacts, but this occupant motion could not be reproduced in the laboratory.

The *vehicle seat* influences occupant motion in rear impacts. Though vehicle seats must pass certain minimum standards, there are vast differences in properties. Passenger car seats have a cantilever seat back with a fixed or adjustable head restraint. The seat back height and the head to head restraint distance varies considerably. Seat backs can be stiff or compliant, depending on the nature of the cushioning and the construction of the seat back frame and recline mechanism. Seats with a recline mechanism usually have a ratchet mechanism on the outboard side of the seat cushion/seat back junction. The inboard side is pinned in place. Seats that have been in service for an extended time, or seats in vehicles that have had a significant rear impact, will often warp or twist owing to the differing support on the inboard and outboard sides.

Seat and bumper types have influence on occupant head motion in rear impacts of equal severity. Vehicle motion was recorded with a fifth wheel and force transducers in a rigid collision barrier. Occupant motion was recorded with a biaxial accelerometer fixed with head gear to a point forward and above the right ear of the same male volunteer seated facing forward in the right front seat of each vehicle. Head accelerations were measured in the sagittal plane. Head gear repositioning between tests was highly repeatable, thus eliminating any errors associated with accelerometer placement. The position of the accelerometer was not critical, and no attempt was made to resolve the head accelerations to the head center of mass, because it was not the purpose of the tests to measure absolute head acceleration, only to compare head acceleration among the four passenger cars. Each seat was of the cantilever design with a recline mechanism.

Figure 7 shows a typical vehicle and head acceleration trace at 6.5 km/h ΔV. Note the time lag between the vehicle motion and the head motion. This time lag, which exists regardless of bumper type, means that the bumper does not influence head motion for a given change of velocity at impact. Head acceleration traces are the magnitude of vertical and horizontal accelerations. Vehicles with firmer seat cushioning may produce greater head acceleration peaks for a given ΔV impact.

In *frontal impacts*, the upper and lower body move forward relative to the vehicle, the amount depending on the presence or absence of a seat belt, the severity of the collision, and the friction between the occupant and seat, which depends on seat upholstery and the occupant's clothing but not on the occupant's weight. If the severity is high enough, the head generally moves forward, then downward as the chest is arrested by the torso belt. At very low severities, motion can be resisted by muscle action,

FIGURE 7. Vehicle and head acceleration in minor staged rear impacts at approximately 6.5 km/h ΔV. The vehicle had foam bumper and adjustable head restraint.

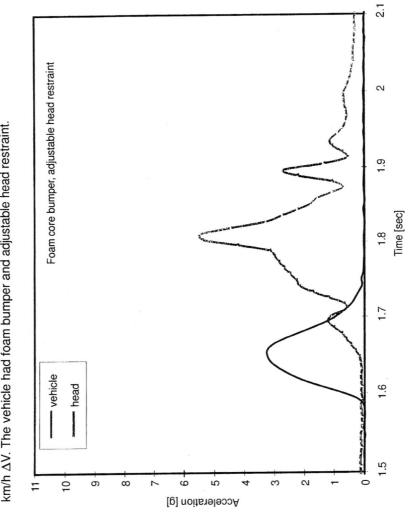

Foam core bumper, adjustable head restraint

particularly by the driver who can perceive the imminent collision and grip the steering wheel. At severities around 10 km/h ΔV or less, the seat belt's influence is somewhat redundant. For high seat cushion/clothing friction combinations [e.g., denim on cloth upholstery] seat belt loads near zero have been observed for male drivers at that impact severity. Lower friction combinations [e.g., synthetic clothing, leather upholstery] may allow enough forward slide at this severity for even a restrained occupant to make knee to dash contact, though the contact is mild.

In *lateral impacts collisions*, the lateral velocity of the target vehicle rapidly goes from steady state to peak then back to steady state, as a result of tire friction in the sliding direction. In minor lateral impacts the sideways movement of the vehicle, and of the occupants hips, may be limited to only a few centimeters. The amount of sideways motion depends in part on the road conditions: high traction [dry pavement] conditions result in less severe motion than low traction [ice or snow] conditions. In good traction conditions, the target vehicle in a minor lateral collision moves sideways beneath the occupant, then stops. In human volunteer tests, it has been observed that the torso, head and neck move as a unit, so that little stress is applied to the neck.

In *side-swipe collisions*, the two vehicles are nearly parallel as one vehicle scrapes along the side of the other. The faster of the two vehicles experiences a long duration frontal impact, and the slower vehicle experiences a long duration rear impact. The vehicles also will experience some small lateral accelerations. If there is no snagging between the vehicles, then the accelerations may be comparable to vehicle accelerations that can be experienced in emergency driving maneuvers. If there is snagging, which may occur at door and fender seems or ends of bumpers, then there will be a more significant impact whose acceleration pulse resembles a front or rear impact. The consequent occupant motions are those associated with front or rear impacts.

Human tolerance to minor impacts is better understood due to a growing body of data from staged collisions. Many of the tests involved passenger vehicles, some tests involved impact sleds with various seating and restraint arrangements and one series involved amusement park bumper cars. These results from 252 staged collisions in which a volunteer was seated in the struck vehicle are shown in Figure 8 for rear-end, front-end and lateral collisions. (3,8,9,10,12,13,14,15,16). The tolerance for symptoms is reached at much lower severity in the rear impact than in the frontal or lateral impact. In all types the symptoms were either non-existent, or ranged from neck and headaches that lasted a few minutes to a few

FIGURE 8. Summary of human volunteer data. Note different icons for males and females.

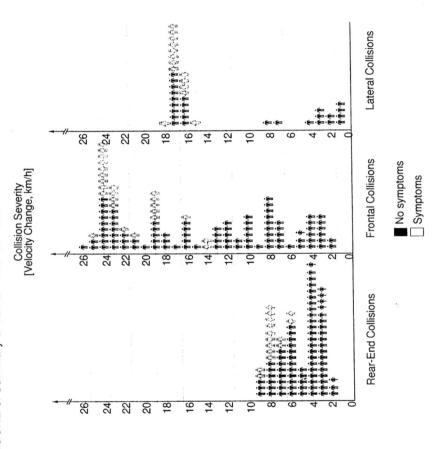

Collision Severity
[Velocity Change, km/h]

Rear-End Collisions

Frontal Collisions

Lateral Collisions

■ No symptoms
□ Symptoms

days. In the lateral impacts there were occasional reports of hip pain, and of neck pain that had delays to onset up to 24 hours.

These studies have focused on a correlation between severity and symptoms. Among other influential factors besides severity are age, gender, stature, medical history, posture and preparedness. Of the 252 tests, only 13 have involved a female. All of the volunteers have been healthy, with no known significant pre-existing medical conditions. In almost all tests, the subjects have adopted a posture representative of driving a vehicle, typically sitting erect with a properly adjusted seat belt and head restraint. In all tests the volunteer subjects were aware of the impending impact, though in rear impacts removal of visual and audio stimuli kept the subjects unaware of the precise time of impact, and most subjects attempted to maintain a relaxed muscle tone while awaiting the impact. The significance of these variables, particularly posture [head turned compared to forward looking], has not been studied extensively in controlled tests.

REFERENCES

1. Bailey M, King D, Rommilly D, Thomson R: Characterization of automobile bumper components for low speed impacts. Proc Can Multidisciplinary Road Safety Conf VII: 1991.

2. King D, Siegmund G, Bailey M: Automobile bumper behavior in low-speed impacts. SAE 930211.

3. Siegmund G, Bailey M, King D: Characteristics of specific automobile bumpers in low-velocity impacts. SAE 940916.

4. Griffin M: Evaluation of vibration with respect to human response. SAE 860047.

5. Bailey M, Wong B, Lawrence, J: Data and methods for estimating the severity of minor impacts. SAE 950352.

6. Nagel D, Manning J, Chadwick C, Cronin R, Gould R: Human tolerance data from "real life" motor vehicle accidents. Amer Assoc for Automotive Med: 16th Conf, 1972.

7. Severy DM, Mathewson J, Bechtol M: Controlled automobile rear-end collisions, an investigation of related engineering and medical phenomena, Can Services Med: 727-759, Nov 1955.

8. Szabo T, Welcher J, Anderson R, et al.: Human occupant kinematic responses to low-speed rear-end impacts. SAE 940532.

9. McConnell W, Howard R, Guzman H, et al.: Analysis of human test subject kinematic responses to low velocity rear end impacts. SAE 930889.

10. Scott M, McConnell W, Guzman H, et al.: Comparison of human and ATD head kinematics during low-speed rear-end impacts. SAE 930094.

11. Snider A, Dance M: Emergency locking retractor performance in low speed direct rear-end collisions. Can Assoc of Technical Accident Investigators and Reconstructionists: August 1990.

12. Siegmund G, Williamson P: Speed change [ΔV] of amusement park bumper cars. Can Multidisciplinary Motor Vehicle Safety Conference VIII: 1993.

13. Chandler R. Christian, R: Crash testing of humans in automobile seats. SAE 700361.

14. Glenn T: Anthropomorphic dummy and human volunteer tests of advanced and/or passive belt restraint systems. SAE 740579.

15. Ewing C, Thomas D: Human head and neck response to impact acceleration. Naval Aerospace Med Res Lab: August 1972.

16. Zaborowski A: Human tolerance to lateral impact with lap belt only. SAE 640843.

Low Speed Rear Impact Collisions: In Search of an Injury Threshold

Arthur C. Croft

SUMMARY. From a review of current literature, it would appear that, a. a significant transfer of energy occurs in low speed rear impact collisions [LoSRICs], b. the kinematics of these accidents is quite complex and probably explains the unique risk to this form of trauma, c. a large portion of persons injured in LoSRICs continue to suffer from residuals of those injuries, d. the prevalence of chronic symptoms of these injuries in the U.S. has been estimated at 1-12%, e. the threshold for injury has not yet been adequately investigated to allow reasonable conclusions to be made about the universe of persons at risk of injury from LoSRIC–particularly considering the multitude of other complicating variables, such as second collisions, disparity in sizes of involved vehicles, etc. Therefore, the threshold for injury at the current time remains largely unknown, and there does not appear to be any scientifically or empirically sound basis for reliably gauging injury potential from vehicle property damage or other aspects of the crash, such as the speed of the involved vehicles. *[Article copies available from The Haworth Document Delivery Service: 1-800-342-9678. E-mail address: getinfo@haworth.com]*

KEYWORD. Whiplash, low speed rear impact collision, cervical acceleration/deceleration injury

---

Arthur C. Croft, DC, MS, FACO, is Director, Spine Research Institute, San Diego, and Assistant Adjunct Professor, Los Angeles College of Chiropractic.

Address correspondence to: Arthur C. Croft, DC, Spine Research Institute, 402-5030 Camino de La Siesta, San Diego, CA 92108-3119.

[Haworth co-indexing entry note]: "Low Speed Rear Impact Collisions: In Search of an Injury Threshold." Croft, Arthur C. Co-published simultaneously in *Journal of Musculoskeletal Pain* [The Haworth Medical Press, an imprint of The Haworth Press, Inc.] Vol. 4, No. 4, 1996, pp. 39-46; and: *Musculoskeletal Pain Emanating from the Head and Neck: Current Concepts in Diagnosis, Management and Cost Containment* [ed: Murray E. Allen] The Haworth Medical Press, an imprint of The Haworth Press, Inc., 1996, pp. 39-46. Single or multiple copies of this article are available from The Haworth Document Delivery Service [1-800-342-9678, 9:00 a.m. - 5:00 p.m. [EST]. E-mail address: getinfo@haworth.com].

39

INTRODUCTION

Since the first automobiles appeared on American roads, clinicians have ministered to those claiming injury from low speed rear impact collisions [LoSRICs]. Although great strides have been made in our understanding of this condition, it remains a controversial topic.

The term "whiplash," which is frequently applied to the congeries of resulting and often bewildering symptoms, was coined in the 1920s, but has recently given way to more kinematically descriptive terminology, such as "cervical acceleration/deceleration" [CAD] injury (1). In this paper, these terms will be synonymous, although the reader should remember that some authors define whiplash as any neck injury resulting from any automobile collision.

Full Scale Crash Testing

The nature of the injury resulting from LoSRICs is primarily soft tissue and, as a result of the difficulties encountered in demonstrating objective lesions, coupled with the common association with litigation, CAD injuries have suffered a rather undeserved poor reputation within the clinical community. In the 1950s Severy et al. (2,3) developed a hypothesis that human occupants in such collisions may be exposed to accelerations of equal or higher magnitude than that of the struck vehicle itself. This hypothesis was verified in crash tests using a human volunteer and an anthropometric dummy in which the acceleration of the volunteer's head was measured at 2.5 times that of the vehicle during 12.8 km/h collisions. Later criticisms that this model was no longer valid in the context of modern vehicles equipped with newer safety devices, such as seatbelts, shoulder harnesses, head restraints, and bumper isolators [or other energy dissipating bumper systems], was subsequently dampened when Navin et al. (4) conducted similar experiments with late model Volkswagens using a pendulum impactor and Hybrid II anthropometric dummies. They demonstrated not only the same temporal relationships found by the Severy group, but similar energy relationships as well. The basic elements of the Severy et al. CAD model, therefore, remain valid.

McConnell et al. (5) have more recently evaluated the human response to LoSRICs in the two through five mph range. Their four test subjects, which included the researchers themselves, were described as "robustly healthy" adult males. All were subjected to multiple impacts at low speed. The authors described the detailed kinematic results of their research, including observations not previously noted, and concluded that 8 km/h [5 mph] impacts were the threshold for mild cervical strain injury.

Low speed rear impact collisions were also the subject of investigation by Szabo et al. (6) who performed six crash tests using five human subjects [again, the researchers] at 8 km/h. In this project the subjects were of both genders. Complex kinematic results were reported. Four of the subjects underwent pre- and post-impact magnetic resonance imaging [MRI] examination. Other than transient symptoms, no long term physical complaints were reported and there were no significant MRI findings. Among the conclusions, the authors reported that their study supported the premise that restrained occupants of rear impact collisions at speeds of 8 km/h or less are unlikely to sustain injury.

Rosenbluth and Hicks (7) have attempted to develop a system to allow investigators to quantify collision severity by first evaluating impact artifacts [such as isolator travel] and then calculating a barrier equivalent velocity [BEV; also referred to as equivalent barrier speed, or EBS]. Occupant stress and likelihood of injury can also be calculated by their model, they claim.

OUTCOME STUDIES

While engineers have struggled to understand the complex mechanics of LoSRICs, other researchers have followed groups of CAD-injured occupants through time in hope of developing reliable and valid models for estimating prognosis. The earliest of these studies was that of Gotten (8) who found that at one year follow-up, 46% continued to have physical complaints related to the auto accident. This report was followed by one from Macnab (9) who reported that at least 45% of his patients were symptomatic more than two years after settlement of their claims. Several subsequent studies reported the long range percentages of symptomaticity (10-21), ranging from a low outlyer of 12% to two of the more recent studies that followed patients for much longer periods [more than 10 years]. Both found that 86% continued to have complaints, confirming the often doleful outcome for these injuries. However, precise interpretation of most of these studies is hampered by selection bias, difficulty in comparability between groups, and other forms of methodological error (22).

INCIDENCE AND PREVALENCE

Accurate figures for the incidence of CAD injury from LoSRICs are not available. However, in 1971 the National Safety Council estimated that there were nearly four million rear end impact accidents in the United

States of America [U.S.] with about one million resulting injuries (23). In the U.S. a National Accident Sampling System is in place and compiles data from regionally selected hospitals and police agencies in an effort to estimate the magnitude of various types of accidents (24). While accurate for the higher end of the injury spectrum, where victims are seen either at hospitals or by police, these estimating systems generally underreport the less severe injuries since police are not usually present at the accident scene and since victims frequently do not report to emergency rooms for treatment. Kahane (25), for example, has reported that 55% of CAD injuries are not accounted for in police reports.

Incidence rates for CAD injury have been reported in Denmark (26) at 28/100,000. The authors of the *Quebec Task Force Monograph* (27) reported an incidence of 70/100,000 for Quebec and compared that figure to reports from New Zealand [13/100,000], Australia [106/100,000], and Saskatchewan [700/100,000]. The latter rate appears most comparable with the U.S. rate, based on interpretation of the previously mentioned data.

The prevalence of patients suffering from long term residual symptoms of CAD injury has not been carefully studied. One study estimated that 6-12% of the U.S. population may be affected (28). Barnsley et al. (29) have estimated this figure more conservatively at 1%. Even at 1%, however, the magnitude of the problem is stunning since, in theory, the condition is largely preventable. A portion of these injuries might be prevented through safe driver education programs and the development of intelligent highway/vehicle systems designed to warn drivers of stopped or slow moving vehicles in their path. In addition, the crashworthiness of passenger vehicles can probably be improved through the development of seat backs, head restraints, and bumper systems designed to reduce occupant acceleration during rear impact crashes.

DISCUSSION

Of the studies mentioned, most are problematic to some degree. In most of the full scale crash tests involving human volunteers, brakes were not used, thereby allowing the struck vehicle to free-wheel after impact. The volunteers were aware of the impending collision and were seated in an upright and straight forward posture with properly fastened restraints. In real world collisions occupants may have brakes applied at the time of impact and secondary collisions may occur—both conditions accentuate the deceleration phase of the injury. Many have their heads turned at the time of impact or are seated in out-of-position postures. These conditions are also associated with a greater risk of injury. Differences in the relative sizes of the striking and struck vehicles is an important issue, but all crash testing to date has utilized relatively similar sized vehicles. Epidemiological research has consistently demonstrated that females are more frequently injured in these accidents than males, and also have greater long term disability. Yet only one of the studies mentioned has employed female subjects.

Although the Szabo et al. (6) and McConnell et al. (5) papers made important contributions to our pool of knowledge, some of their conclusions regarding the potential for injury in these collisions is not justified on a scientific basis because: 1. females were not used in the McConnell et al. (5) study and, as a result, they can not extrapolate their findings to female occupants, 2. all subjects had knowledge of the impending impact [the use of ear plugs to eliminate this problem, as reported by the authors, is not valid], 3. the use of follow-up MRI in the Szabo et al. (6) study is not a valid outcome measure for the universe of expected findings [which include long term degenerative changes] since the waiting period between pre- and post-MRI was shorter than one in which we would expect to see degenerative changes develop, 4. both studies involved very small samples of healthy volunteers which did not represent the entire population of persons at risk. Their conclusions, therefore, can not be extrapolated to, for example, the elderly, the very young, persons with advanced degenerative changes in their spines, persons with other pre-existing spinal conditions, etc. Also problematic is the method of outcome assessment. Volunteers were examined after the crash tests and again several months later. Due to the well known latency of degenerative changes following CAD types of exposure, a more rigorous examination and longer follow-up would seem warranted. The other aforementioned variables that were excluded from study [out-of-position-effect, etc.] further limit the conclusions that can be drawn from these studies.

Since most of these variables have been shown to affect outcome, and since most were not evaluated by or controlled for by the authors mentioned, there appears to be no scientific basis for the broad conclusion that 8 km/h is the threshold for cervical strain injury in LoSRICs unless we limit the statement to robustly healthy adult males, aware of the impending impact, and [in the majority of instances] using proper restraint equipment, while seated squarely in the seat. If we were to consider the entire population at risk, in combination with the multitude of known risk variables, we would most likely find that the threshold for injury for some individuals, and under certain conditions, is probably lower than 8 km/h.

Crash tests have shown that when two vehicles equipped with 8 km/h rated bumpers collide at speeds as high as 16 km/h, property damage may be negligible. Therefore, the information provided by McConnell et al. (5), while of great academic interest, leaves us wanting for a practical application. For example, a collision can conceivably exceed their reported threshold for injury [notwithstanding the potential error of this estimate] by a factor of two, with little or no measurable resulting vehicle damage from which to gauge the extent of soft tissue injury. Nevertheless, the 8 km/h threshold theory has not been lost on those who routinely attempt to insulate themselves against personal injury claims by arguing that a lack of property damage is tantamount to a lack of soft tissue injury. Yet there is no scientific basis for such a conclusion. Collateral arguments suggest that persons engaged in litigation suffer from accident neurosis or litigation neurosis. Careful investigation, however, has failed to validate the constructs of either of these conditions (30).

A common empirical observation, made by those who treat these patients frequently, is that the extent of injuries to two occupants of the same vehicle often varies widely–largely as a result of the great diversity of human variables, such as preparedness, body type, position, pre-existing condition, muscle strength, etc. In many cases, one occupant will be injured when another is not. This observation alone should be adequate to discourage the practice of calculating the occupant's injury potential based only on assessment of impact magnitude. Such information should not be considered the final truth of a case, but rather used as a guide by the clinical professions in dealing with trauma and its consequences.

CONCLUSION

On balance, it would appear that a. a significant transfer of energy occurs in LoSRICs, b. the kinematics are quite complex and probably explain the unique risk in this form of trauma, c. a portion of persons injured in LoSRICs continues to suffer from residuals of those injuries, d. the prevalence of chronic symptoms of these injuries in the U.S. has been estimated at 1-12%, e. the threshold for injury has not yet been adequately investigated to allow reasonable conclusions to be made about the universe of persons at risk of injury from LoSRIC–particularly considering the multitude of other complicating variables [such as second collisions, disparity in sizes of involved vehicles, etc.]. Therefore, the threshold for injury at the current time can roughly be set at 8 km/h for otherwise healthy males, but is unknown for other groups, and f. there does not appear to be any scientifically or empirically sound basis for reliably gauging injury potential from vehicle property damage or other aspects of the crash, such as the speed of the involved vehicles.

We should continue to investigate kinematic models of LoSRICs using anthropometric human surrogates that provide the best fit for recorded human responses to low speed impacts. Dummy studies will allow engineers to design bumper and frame systems, safety harnesses, head restraints, and seatbacks that will reduce the potential for injury in accidents that can't otherwise be averted. More accurate determination of human injury thresholds, unfortunately, will require testing of humans rather than dummies. At the same time we must attempt to develop a more comprehensive model for the prediction of human injury based on a number of variables, such as pre-existing spondylosis, that are already known to have a significant effect on outcome. More work also is needed in the investigation of all other risk factors that either predispose to injury or give rise to poor outcome. Finally, clinical researchers must continue to develop treatment paradigms that will prove most effective for the wide range of clinical conditions that result from CAD injury.

REFERENCES

1. Croft AC: Biomechanics. In Foreman SM, Croft AC (eds), Whiplash Injuries: The Cervical Acceleration/Deceleration Syndrome (2nd edition), Baltimore, Williams & Wilkins, 1995, p3.

2. Severy DM, Mathewson JH, Bechtol CO: Controlled automobile rear-end collisions, an investigation of related engineering and mechanical phenomenon. Can Services Med J 11:727-758, 1955.

3. Severy DM, Mathewson JH: Automobile barrier and rear-end collision performance. Paper presented at the Society of Automotive Engineers summer meeting, Atlantic City, NJ, June 8-13, 1958.

4. Navin FPD, Romilly DP: An investigation into vehicle and occupant response subjected to low-speed rear impacts. Proceedings of the Multidisciplinary Road Safety Conference VI, Fredericton, New Brunswick, June 5-7, 1989.

5. McConnell WH, Howard RP, Guzman HM, et al.: Analysis of human test subject kinematic responses to low velocity rear end impacts. SAE 9308889.

6. Szabo TJ, Welcher JB, Anderson RD, Rice MM, Ward JA, Paulo LR, Carpenter NJ: Human occupant response to low speed rear-end impacts. SAE 940532.

7. Rosenbluth W, Hicks L: Evaluating low-speed rear-end impact severity and resultant occupant stress parameters. J Forensic Sciences 1393-1424, Nov, 1994.

8. Gotten N: Survey of one hundred cases of whiplash injury after settlement of litigation. JAMA 162(9):865-867, 1956.

9. Macnab I: Acceleration injuries of the cervical spine. J Bone Joint Surg 46A(8):1797-1799, 1964.

10. Hohl M: Soft tissue injuries of the neck in automobile accidents: factors influencing prognosis. J Bone Joint Surg 56A(8):1675-1682, 1974.

11. Ellertsson AB, Sigurjusson K, Thorsteinsson T: Clinical and radiographic study of 100 cases of whiplash injury. Acth Neurol Scand (Suppl) 67:269, 1978.

12. Norris SH, Watt I: The prognosis of neck injuries resulting from rear-end vehicle collisions. J Bone Joint Surg 65B(5):608-611, 1983.

13. Ebbs SR, Beckly DE, Hammonds JC, Teasdale C: Incidence and duration of neck pain among patients injured in car accidents. Br Med J 292:94-95, 1986.

14. Deans GT, Magalliard JN, Kerr M, Rutherford WH: Neck sprain–a major cause of disability following car accidents. Injury 18:10-12, 1987.

15. Maimaris C, Barnes MR, Allen MJ: 'Whiplash injuries' of the neck: a retrospective study. Injury 19(5):393-396, 1988.

16. Pearce JMS: Whiplash injury: a reappraisal. J Neurol Neurosurg Psychiatr 52:1329-1331, 1989.

17. Hodgson SP, Grundy M: Whiplash injuries: their long-term prognosis and its relationship to compensation. Neuro Orthop 7:88-99, 1989.

18. Hildingson C, Toolanen G: Outcome after soft-tissue injury of the cervical spine. Acta Orthop Scand 61(4):357-359, 1990.

19. Watkinson A, Gargan MG, Bannister GC: Prognostic factors in soft tissue injuries of the cervical spine. Injury 22(4):307-309, 1991.

20. Parmar HV, Raymakers R: Neck injuries from rear impact road traffic accidents: prognosis in persons seeking compensation. Injury 24(2):75-78, 1993.

21. Robinson DD, Cassar-Pullicino VN: Acute neck sprain after road traffic accident: a long-term clinical and radiological review. Injury 24(2):79-82, 1993.

22. Croft AC: Proposed classification of cervical acceleration/deceleration (CAD) injuries with a review of prognostic research. Palmer J Research 1(1): 10-21, 1994.

23. National Safety Council. Accident Facts. Chicago, National Safety Council, 1971, p 47.

24. National Accident Sampling System: 1986–a report on traffic crashes and injuries in the United States. U.S. Department of Transportation, NHTSA.

25. Kahane CJ: An evaluation of head restraints–FMVSS 202. NHTSA Technical Report DOT HS-806-108, Feb, 1982.

26. Juhl M, Kjaergaard S: Cervical spine injuries. Epidemiological investigation. Medical and social consequences. 6th International IRCOBI Conference, Salon-de-Provence, France, Sep 8-10, 1981.

27. Spitzer WO, Skovron ML, Salmi LR, Cassidy JD, Duranceau J, Suissa S, Zeiss E: Scientific monograph of the Quebec task force on whiplash-associated disorders: redefining "whiplash" and its management. Spine Supplement (April 15) 20(8S), 1995.

28. Croft AC: Whiplash: The Epidemic (4th edition). San Diego, Spine Research Institute of San Diego.

29. Barnsley L, Lord S, Bogduk N: Whiplash injury. Pain 58:283-307, 1994.

30. Croft AC: The case against litigation neurosis in mild brain injuries and cervical acceleration/deceleration trauma. J Neuromusculoskeletal Syst 1(4):149-155, 1993.

The Effect of Accident Mechanisms and Initial Findings on the Long-Term Outcome of Whiplash Injury

Bogdan P. Radanov
Matthias Sturzenegger

SUMMARY. Objectives: To analyze the relationship between somatic, radiological and neuropsychological findings and features of the accident mechanisms assessed early after trauma and long-term outcome after whiplash injury.

Findings: Patients who remained symptomatic during two years of trauma were older, showed more rotated or inclined head position at the time of impact, had higher prevalence of pre-traumatic headache, scored higher on ratings of initial neck pain and headache, dis-

---

Bogdan P. Radanov, MD, is Associate Professor, Department Psychiatry, University of Berne, Switzerland, and Head of Psychiatric Consultation and Liaison Service, University General Hospital, Berne. Matthias Sturzenegger, MD, is Professor, Department Psychiatry, University Berne, Switzerland.

Address correspondence to: Bogdan P. Radanov, Department Psychiatry, University of Berne, Inselspital, CH-3010 Berne, Switzerland.

This study is an abbreviated version of previously published work (7) and was supported by the Swiss National Science Foundation [project number 3. 883-0.88] and the Swiss Accident Insurance Company [Schweizerische Unfallversicherungsanstalt], regional agency Berne.

[Haworth co-indexing entry note]: "The Effect of Accident Mechanisms and Initial Findings on the Long-Term Outcome of Whiplash Injury." Radanov, Bogdan P., and Matthias Sturzenegger. Co-published simultaneously in *Journal of Musculoskeletal Pain* [The Haworth Medical Press, an imprint of The Haworth Press, Inc.] Vol. 4, No. 4, 1996, pp. 47-59; and: *Musculoskeletal Pain Emanating from the Head and Neck: Current Concepts in Diagnosis, Management and Cost Containment* [ed: Murray E. Allen] The Haworth Medical Press, an imprint of The Haworth Press, Inc., 1996, pp. 47-59. Single or multiple copies of this article are available from The Haworth Document Delivery Service [1-800-342-9678, 9:00 a.m. - 5:00 p.m. [EST]. E-mail address: getinfo@haworth.com].

played a greater variety of symptoms, had a higher incidence of symptoms of radicular deficit and higher average scores on a multiple symptom analysis, and showed more osteoarthrosis on x-ray. These same patients, in addition, on testing showed impaired well-being and deficient attentional processing, and had more concern with regard to long-term suffering and disability.

Conclusions: These findings essentially support the view that a poor outcome in the long-term after whiplash injury is primarily related to its initial severity. *[Article copies available from The Haworth Document Delivery Service: 1-800-342-9678. E-mail address: getinfo@ haworth.com]*

KEYWORDS. Whiplash, prospective, longitudinal outcome

INTRODUCTION

In order to overcome limitations from previous reports with whiplash patients best summarized in the *Scientific Monograph of the Quebec Task Force on Whiplash-Associated Disorders* (1) present research was designed as a multidisciplinary study to investigate patients referred from primary care within the shortest time of injury according to a strict injury-definition and to follow-up these individuals during 24 months.

PATIENTS AND METHODS

As reported in several previous publications (2,3,4,5,6,7,8) a non-selected sample was obtained by announcing this study in the *Swiss Medical Journal* and repeatedly distributing letters to primary care physicians in our catchment area. Physicians were asked to refer patients within the shortest possible interval after whiplash injury. We adopted the definition proposed by Hirsch et al. (9) that common whiplash is a trauma causing cervical musculo-ligamental sprain or strain due to hyperflexion/hyperextension. In addition, diagnosis in our study excludes fractures or dislocations of the cervical spine, head injury or alteration of consciousness. Furthermore, in order to avoid trans-cultural differences in illness behavior we considered only patients with German as their native language. Patients with previous neurological deficits or injuries to other parts of the body were also excluded. Finally, patients older than 55 years were also excluded [because of norms on neuropsychological testing].

As detailed previously (4,5,6,7,8) over the sampling period of two years, 164 patients were referred of which 27 failed to meet the inclusion criteria and 20 patients dropped out during follow-up. The investigated sample consisted of 117 patients [mean age = 30.7 ± 9.6 years, range 19-51 years, 58% women, all injured in automobile accidents and fully covered by accident insurance*].

Patients were initially investigated on an average of 7.2 ± 4.2 days of trauma and follow-up examinations were performed at three [T2], six [T3], twelve [T4] and 24 months [T5]. During the follow-up period patients' treatment was the responsibility of the referring physicians, who were sent detailed information on all aspects of each investigation, however, without treatment recommendations from our group (7). Patients who had fully recovered at the six-months examination [i.e., did not complain of any trauma-related symptoms] were released from the study, but were interviewed by phone after two years. However, there was a possibility for these patients to be rereferred if any symptoms re-occurred (7).

As reported previously (2,3,4,5,6,7) examinations included:

1. Semistructured interviews which at baseline assessed features of accident mechanisms, patients' assessment of accident, initial subjective complaints and the interval between injury and the onset of neck pain and headache as well as the latency to display initial symptoms (6,7). Attention was given to previous cervico-cephalic trauma and history of headache including its type (9-12). Injury mechanism was evaluated by documenting impact to the car, patient's position in the car, use of head rests and seat-belts and the head position at the time of impact (7). A symptom-score was calculated for each patient at the initial examination using posterior neck pain, headache, shoulder pain, back pain, anterior neck pain, dysphagia, vertigo, unsteadiness, visual disturbance, tinnitus, symptoms of radicular irritation, and symptoms of myelopathy [each presented symptom was given a score of 1]. At follow-ups patients subjective complaints were documented according to a structured interview scheme (7):
2. Complete neurological and physical examinations were performed at baseline and at T3, T4 and T5. Based on initial findings the fol-

---

*According to the Swiss Accident Insurance System, if the patient loses time from work because of injury, the patient receives a proportional amount of salary regardless of liability. Certification of disability is the task of the treating physician. The system does not provide compensation for non-economic loss such as pain or suffering. If permanent disability is expected [i.e., no therapeutic measure is likely to improve patients health status] a final disability assessment is initiated. This usually happens several months after the accident.

lowing grading system of severity of injury was applied (7,8): Grade 1: symptoms only; Grade 2: symptoms and restricted neck movement; Grade 3: symptoms, restricted neck movement and evidence of objective neurological loss;

3. Cervical spine x-rays at baseline included antero-posterior, lateral, right and left oblique as well as lateral views in flexion and extension, the antero-posterior view in lateral inclination and the transoral view of the Dens (6,7,8);

4. Self-ratings of initial neck pain and headache intensity [using a scale from 0 = no pain, to 10 points = maximal pain] (2,3,4,5,6,7,8) were assessed at all investigations;

5. Patients' personal and family history and current psychosocial disposition (7,10,11,12);

6. A set of formal psychological (2,3,4,5,6,7,8) and cognitive (3,5,6,7) tests was performed at all investigations and included: a. Personality traits, examined by the Freiburg Personality Inventory (10) as reported previously (2,5,6,7); b. Self-rated well-being was assessed by the Well-being scale [WBS] (11) using parallel versions at follow-ups; c. Change in trauma-related cognitive ability was evaluated using the Cognitive Failures Questionnaire [CFQ] (12); d. A series of formal tests of attention including: the Digit Span (13), Corsi block tapping (14), the Trail Making Test, Parts A and B [TMT-A and TMT-B] (15), the Number Connection Test [NCT] (16), and the Paced Auditory Serial Addition Task [PASAT] (17).

At the two-year examination, subjects were divided into symptomatic [persistence of symptoms] and asymptomatic groups [completely recovered]. Employing the χ^2 test for dichotomous variables and Mann-Whitney U-test for interval-scaled variables [e.g., scores on different tests], the two groups were compared with respect to initial findings from the baseline examination. Differences between baseline and the two year scores of pain intensity and psychological variables of patients from the symptomatic group was assessed using the Wilcoxon matched-pair signed-ranks test. The course of cognitive and psychological functioning was analysed during follow-up using scores of symptomatic and asymptomatic groups.

RESULTS

Fifty-one patients [44%] after three, 36 [30%] after six, 28 [24%] after twelve, and 21 patients [18%] after 24 months, suffered from persistent injury related symptoms [symptomatic group]. Symptomatic patients were older [P < 0.03] but groups did not differ regarding gender or educational attainment. Comparing the symptomatic patients after two years with those who had completely recovered with regard to initial findings the following observations appeared relevant [Table 1]: Symptomatic patients had significantly more rotated or inclined head position at the time of impact, and reported a greater variety of subjective complaints at the initial examination. In the same group significant differences were found regarding prevalence of pre-traumatic headache, and initial pain ratings for headache [P < 0.004] and neck pain [P < 0.008], the latter two remaining high over the follow-up period [Figure 1]. Furthermore this group had significantly more symptoms of radicular-type deficit [*non-radicular symptoms*] which, however, could not be objectively shown during clinical neurologic examination. In addition, the symptomatic group showed higher average scores on multiple symptom analysis and significantly more indications of osteoarthrosis on initial x-ray [P < 0.017]. Regarding initially assessed aspects of psychosocial stress or scales from personality inventory, there were no significant differences between the groups. The symptomatic group scored significantly higher on the WBS [P < 0.023] and performed significantly worse on NCT [P < 0.0001], TMT-A [P < 0.026] and TMT-B [P < 0.012] and PASAT [P < 0.023], whereas there was no significant difference regarding the CFQ [see Figure 2].

The apparent difference with regard to attentional functioning between groups at T1, T2 and T3 [Figure 2], showed no statistically significant differences when comparing groups using multivariate analysis of variance [MANOVA] with age and medication as covariates.

When comparing the initial [T1] with the final examination [T5] in the symptomatic group the following findings deserve mention: 1. Significant differences were found on the NCT [Z = − 3.49, P < 0.001], TMT-B [Z = − 2.01, P < 0.05] and PASAT [Z = − 3.13, P < 0.002] where, on average, an improvement was found; 2. No significant differences between T1 and T5 were found on CFQ [Z = − 1.66, P = 0.09], depression scale [Z = − 0.08, P = 0.93], openness scale [Z = − 0.69, P = 0.48], neuroticism scale [Z = − 1.03, P = 0.30] and, nervousness scale [Z = − 1.90, P = 0.057]. In contrast significant differences were found on the WBS [Z = − 2.15, P < 0.04] and masculinity scale [Z = − 2.51, P < 0.02] which on average showed an improvement.

DISCUSSION

The present study assessed an essentially non-selected sample of whiplash patients chosen according to clearly defined injury criteria. This and the uniquely comprehensive assessment of patients allows the unbiased

TABLE 1. Findings from the Initial Examination.

ITEMS	Asymptomatic at 2 years N = 96		Symptomatic at 2 years N = 21		P
	N	%	N	%	
Accident-related variables, injury mechanism					
Accident: pure rear-end	33	34	11	52	ns
Accident: frontal	27	28	5	24	ns
Accident: rear-end followed by frontal	22	23	4	19	ns
Accident: other	13	13	2	9	ns
Patient unprepared for accident	70	73	16	76	ns
Head rotated or inclined	27	28	12	57	<.008
Illness or disability worry	25	26	11	52	<.017
Familiarity with symptoms of whiplash injury	47	49	9	43	ns
Initial subjective complaints					
Neck pain	88	92	20	96	ns
Headache	51	53	16	76	ns
Increased fatiguability	50	52	16	76	<.043
Shoulder pain	44	46	13	62	ns
Anxiety with being in car	38	40	14	67	<.023
Sleep disturbances	30	31	16	76	<.0001
Back pain	36	37	9	43	ns
Sensitivity to noise	26	27	8	38	ns
Impaired ability to concentrate	23	24	8	38	ns
Blurred vision	16	17	9	43	<.008
Irritability	18	19	7	33	ns
Dizziness, light-headed	12	12	6	29	ns
Forgetfullness, but no memory loss	10	10	7	33	<.006
Difficulty in swallowing	8	8	2	9	ns
Jugular pain	8	8	1	5	ns
Neurological findings					
Neck muscle tenderness	69	72	18	86	ns
Restricted neck movement	52	54	14	67	ns
Non-radicular symptoms	12	12	5	24	ns
Symptoms of radicular deficit	11	12	6	29	<.043
Symptoms of nerve or brain stem disturbance	28	29	13	62	<.004
Diplopia	2	2	2	9	ns
Oscillopsia	2	2	0	0	ns
Unsteadiness while walking or standing	12	12	6	29	ns
Vertigo	5	5	1	5	ns
Tinnitus	4	4	1	5	ns
Transitory quadraparesis	3	3	2	9	ns
Injury Severity: Grade 1	15	16	2	9	ns
Injury Severity: Grade 2	69	72	18	86	ns
Injury Severity: Grade 3	12	12	1	5	ns
Multiple symptom score	2.9 ± 1.4		3.9 ± 1.9		<.026
Radiological findings					
Misalignment of cervical curvature	46	48	12	57	ns
Signs of degeneration, osteoarthrosis	18	19	9	43	<.017
Psychosocial stress					
Symptoms of childhood emotional deprivations	39	41	7	33	ns
Performance problems in school	19	20	4	19	ns
Dysfunctional family	19	20	5	24	ns
Family history of somatic illness–modeling	37	38	11	52	ns
History of psychological or behavioral problems	24	25	7	33	ns

FIGURE 1. Neck pain and headache self-ratings during follow-up period.

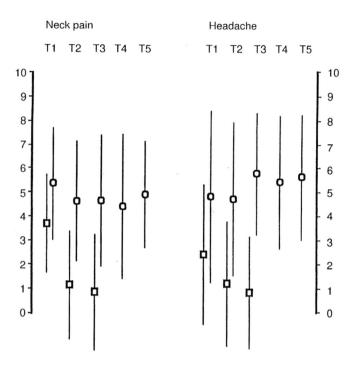

□ patients who remained symtomatic at two years [T5]

□ patients who recovered during follow-up, and were asymptomatic at two years [T5]

evaluation of the consequences of whiplash injury in the long-term. In addition, all patients were injured in automobile accidents, had similar socio-economic and educational backgrounds and were fully covered by accident insurance thus leading to a highly homogeneous sample. Based on the fact that the country-wide insurance scheme provides only for economic loss, bias due to compensation-seeking behavior in this sample is improbable which is, however, an important consideration when comparing results of our study with those of previous studies.

Based on the fact that we investigated an essentially unbiased sample

FIGURE 2. Test of attention, well-being, and self-rated cognitive ability during follow-up period.

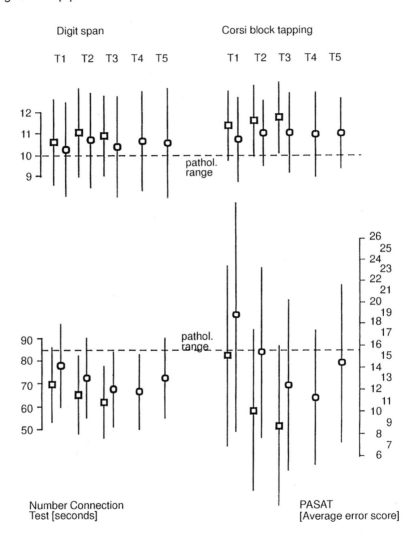

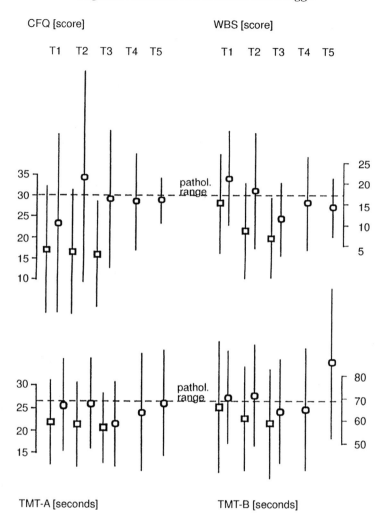

O patients who remained symtomatic at two years [T5]

□ patients who recovered during follow-up being asymptomatic at two years [T5] according to a clear definition, results point towards the notion that whip-lash is a benign condition with a fairly high recovery-rate in which gender or vocational activity do not significantly influence outcome.

The following findings may support the view that symptomatic patients suffered a more severe injury: a greater variety of complaints, higher scoring on pain ratings, a shorter onset latency of initial pain, a significant-ly higher score on multiple symptom analysis, and significantly more ro-tated or inclined head position at the time of impact. The latter makes the cervical spine more susceptible to damage on a biomechanical basis (18,19, 20) and particularly indicates a more severe injury in this group.

The preexisting conditions which appear to favor symptom persistence were; 1. cervical spine osteoarthrosis which was significantly more fre-quent in the symptomatic group and; 2. pre-traumatic headache which showed significantly higher prevalence in the symptomatic group. As discussed earlier (4,6,7) the latter is important for the following reason: the high percentage of patients suffering from pre-traumatic headache in the investigated sample exceeds the prevalence of headache found in the general population (21,22). This may indicate that patients with a history of pre-traumatic headache may be more susceptible to display symptoms following whiplash injury, headache being one of the prominent complaints because of headache triggering based on a pre-formed pattern (4,7).

Consistent with previous results obtained with the same sample during a shorter follow-up period (2,5) psychosocial factors were not of prognostic relevance in the long-term. In accordance with earlier results based on the same sample (3) present findings in addition do not indicate major impair-ment of attentional functioning in whiplash patients in the long-term. There was an average improvement regarding all aspects of attentional function-ing in both groups during the first six months of injury. The subsequently worse performance of symptomatic patients on almost all tests of attention may be explained as follows: a. many of the symptomatic patients used analgesics on a regular basis which may have adverse influence on atten-tion; or b. prolonged suffering from headache of considerably high intensity conceivably impaired attentional function. In addition, scores of headache ratings and scores of tests of attention were paralleled by scores of self-rated cognitive ability thus indicating that these three aspects were closely corre-lated. Worsening of cognitive functioning, as evidenced by changes in test scores, appeared to reflect cognitive impairment due to psychological causes.

The present results favor the usefulness of a comprehensive multidisci-plinary initial assessment of whiplash patients which may help to establish prognosis (23) as well as to understand the course of psychological and cognitive functioning in the long-term as proposed in Figure 3.

FIGURE 3. Factors contributing to development of so-called late whiplash syndrome.

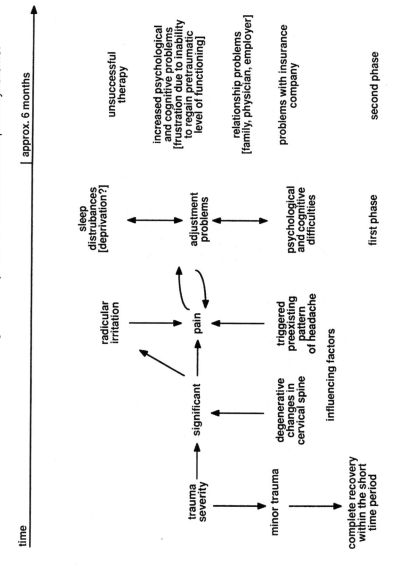

REFERENCES

1. Spitzer WO, Skovron ML, Salmi LR, Cassidy JD, Duranceau J, Suissa S, Zeiss E: Scientific monograph of the Quebec Task Force on whiplash-associated disorders. Best evidence synthesis. Spine 20 (Suppl): S24-33, 1995.

2. Radanov BP, Di Stefano G, Schnidrig A, Ballinari P: Role of psychosocial stress in recovery from common whiplash. Lancet 338: 712-715, 1991.

3. Radanov BP, Di Stefano, Schnidrig A, Sturzenegger M: Cognitive functioning after common whiplash: a controlled follow-up study. Arch Neurol 50: 87-91, 1993.

4. Radanov BP, Sturzenegger M, Di Stefano G, Schnidrig A, Aljinovic M: Factors influencing recovery from headache after common whiplash. BMJ 307: 652-655, 1993.

5. Radanov BP, Di Stefano G, Schnidrig A, Sturzenegger M: Common whiplash—psychosomatic or somatopsychic? J Neurol Neurosurg Psychiatry 57: 486-490, 1994.

6. Radanov BP, Sturzenegger M, Di Stefano G, Schnidrig A: Relationship between early somatic, radiological, cognitive and psychosocial findings and outcome during a one-year follow-up in 117 common whiplash patients. Br J Rheumatol 33: 442-448, 1994.

7. Radanov BP, Sturzenegger M, Di Stefano G: Long-term outcome after whiplash injury—A 2-years follow-up considering features of accident mechanism, somatic, radiological and psychosocial findings. Medicine 74: 281-297, 1995. ©by Williams & Wilkins.

8. Sturzenegger M, Radanov BP, Di Stefano G: The effect of accident mechanisms and initial findings on the long-term course of whiplash injury. J Neurology 242: 443-449, 1995.

9. Hirsch SA, Hirsch PJ, Hiramoto H, Weiss A: Whiplash syndrome: fact or fiction? Orthop Clin N Am 19: 791-795, 1988.

10. Fahrenberg J, Hampel R, Selg H: Das Freiburger Persönlichkietsinventar [FPI] 4th edition, Dr. CJ Hogrefe, Göttingen, 1984.

11. Zerssen vD: Self-rating Scales in the Evaluation of Psychiatric Treatment. In: Methodology in Evaluation of Psychiatric Treatment. Edited by T Helgason. University Press, Cambridge, 1983, 183-204.

12. Broadbent DE, Cooper PF, FitzGerald P, Parkes KR: The cognitive failures questionnaire [CFQ] and its correlates. Br J Clin Psychol 21: 1-16, 1982.

13. Wechsler D: A standardized memory scale for clinical use. J Psychol 19: 87-95, 1945.

14. Milner B: Interhemispheric differences in the localization of psychological processes in man. Br Med Bull 27: 272-277, 1971.

15. Reitan RM: Validity of the trail making test as an indication of organic brain damage. Percept Mot Skills 8: 251-256, 1958.

16. Oswald WD, Roth E: Der Zahlenverbindungstest [ZVT]. 2nd edition. Dr. CJ Hogrefe, Göttingen, 1987.

17. Gronwall D: Paced Auditory Serial Addition Task: A measure of recovery from concussion. Percept Mot Skills 44: 367-373, 1977.

18. Severy DM, Mathewson JH, Bechtol CO: Controlled automobile rear-end collisions, an investigation of related engineering and medical phenomena. Can Serv Med J 11: 727-759, 1955.

19. Wickström J, Martinez J, Rodriguez R: Cervical sprain syndrome and experimental acceleration injuries of the head and neck. In: Proceedings of prevention of highway accidents Symposium. Edited by ML Selzer, PW Gikas, DF Huelke. University of Michigan, Ann Arbor, 1967, 182-187.

20. Tegenthoff M, Malin J-P: Das sogenannte Schleudertrauma der Halswirbelsäule. Anmerkungen aus neurologischer Sicht. Dtsch med Wschr 116: 1030-1034, 1991.

21. Linet MS, Stewart WF, Celentano DD, Ziegler D, Sprecher M: An epidemiologic study of headache among adolescents and young adults. JAMA 261: 2211-2216, 1989.

22. American Psychiatric Association: Diagnostic and Statistical Manual of Mental Disorders. Third edition revised. American Psychiatric Association, Washington DC, 1987, 247-251.

23. Radanov BP, Sturzenegger M: Predicting recovery from common whiplash. Eur Neurol 36: 48-51, 1996.

Cervical Spinal Injuries:
An Autopsy Study of 109 Blunt Injuries

James R. Taylor
Mary M. Taylor

SUMMARY. Objectives: To describe the injuries observed following sagittal sectioning of postmortem cervical spines in 109 blunt trauma fatalities.

Methods: Each spine was carefully removed from skull base to T1, fixed in formalin, deep frozen on dry ice and cut in 2.5 mm sagittal slices on a specially adapted band saw. Sections were viewed using a dissecting microscope.

Results: Spinal injuries were often secondary to head impacts, or to primary accelerations of the torso without head impact. One hundred and two [94%] of the spines showed injuries, more often to the intervertebral joints than to the vertebrae; the majority of the lesions were not visible on postmortem x-rays. The most frequently in-

---

James R. Taylor, MB, ChB, PhD, FAFRM, is Visiting Professor, Australian Neuromuscular Research Institute, and Principal Research Fellow, Royal Perth Hospital, Perth, Australia. Mary M. Taylor, AIMLT, is Research Officer, Royal Perth Hospital.

Address correspondence to: Dr. James R. Taylor, ANRI, Queen Elizabeth II Medical Centre, Nedlands WA 6009 Australia.

Research supported by Medical Research Fund of Western Australia. Facilities for research were provided by Professor B. A. Kakulas and radiological assessment of post mortem radiographs was performed by Dr. Weng Chin.

[Haworth co-indexing entry note]: "Cervical Spinal Injuries: An Autopsy Study of 109 Blunt Injuries." Taylor, James R., and Mary M. Taylor. Co-published simultaneously in *Journal of Musculoskeletal Pain* [The Haworth Medical Press, an imprint of The Haworth Press, Inc.] Vol. 4, No. 4, 1996, pp. 61-79; and: *Musculoskeletal Pain Emanating from the Head and Neck: Current Concepts in Diagnosis, Management and Cost Containment* [ed: Murray E. Allen] The Haworth Medical Press, an imprint of The Haworth Press, Inc., 1996, pp. 61-79. Single or multiple copies of this article are available from The Haworth Document Delivery Service [1-800-342-9678, 9:00 a.m. - 5:00 p.m. (EST). E-mail address: getinfo@haworth.com].

61

jured segments were C1-2, C5-6 and C6-7. In the sub-axial spine, disc and facet injuries were equally common. Spinal cord injuries were seen in 25% of the spines. Nerve root injuries are found in 14% of all the spines and in 33% of those surviving injury for more than two hours; vertebral artery injuries were uncommon.

Conclusion: The neck sprains observed at autopsy, could serve as a guide to the injuries which might be expected in severe "whiplash." Most lesions are to the non-osseous tissues of the joints rather than to the vertebrae and are not readily demonstrable by current imaging techniques. *[Article copies available from The Haworth Document Delivery Service: 1-800-342-9678. E-mail address: getinfo@haworth.com]*

KEYWORDS. Whiplash, spinal trauma, discs, zygapophyseal joints, dorsal root ganglion

INTRODUCTION

Cervical spinal injury is a common consequence of motor vehicle trauma [MVT], falls and blows to the head. In fatal injuries, death usually results from head or chest injuries. Fracture dislocation with spinal cord injury [SCI] is less frequent as the primary cause of death. These severe injuries are readily demonstrated at autopsy but many cervical spinal injuries are not obvious at standard autopsy. A few published studies show that a whole range of "soft tissue injuries" [neck sprain] and fractures can be demonstrated on careful postmortem examination of the cervical spine. These neck injuries are, in themselves, not severe enough to be fatal (1,2,3).

The slender, highly mobile cervical spine, supporting the 4 kilogram head, is vulnerable to injury in sudden accelerations of the head or torso. The gross imbalance in the mass of anterior and posterior neck muscles renders the spine more vulnerable to extension injuries than to flexion injuries (4). In our previous postmortem study of spinal injuries in 385 victims of road trauma, half of all the spinal injuries found were in the cervical spine (5).

The nature and severity of the spinal injury depends on the direction and magnitude of the bending, twisting, shearing, compression or traction forces applied to the neck, and on the strength and compliance of the spinal and surrounding tissues. The most frequent motor vehicle crashes are head-on or rear end collisions, when the force vectors are directed close to the sagittal plane. More than one movement is involved, but the injuries probably reflect the principal force vector.

Neck flexion compresses anterior spinal structures and distracts the posterior elements; extension causes anterior distraction and posterior compression (5,6). In many head impact injuries, axial compression is an important factor (7), when a high percentage of the load is absorbed by the facets. This is due to their 45° orientation and the small vertebral body size (8). Usually, axial compression of the lordotic spine causes buckling into extension.

Cervical spinal injury may result from a primary acceleration of the torso with a non-impact "whiplash" movement of the head and neck, due to its moment of inertia. Alternatively, the injury may result from forced bending of the neck due to a cranio-facial impact (9). Classical accounts of injury, based on clinical and radiological assessment, describe fractures and fracture-dislocations, and focus on injury to the spinal cord (6,10).

Neck sprain or "whiplash" is much more common than fracture dislocation. In most neck sprains, the cervical spine retains a normal alignment, but there are muscular, ligamentous and capsular strains or tears (9). Plain x-rays cannot demonstrate these lesions and magnetic resonance imaging [MRI] can demonstrate some of them (11). Postmortem sectioning can demonstrate the nature of all the lesions (2,5,12).

Clinical series, based on radiological diagnosis (13,14,15) miss most disc lesions and many facet fractures and present an incomplete picture of cervical spinal injuries (16,17). Occasionally, a "widened disc space" (18) or prevertebral soft tissue widening (19) indicates a non-osseous injury. Comparisons of radiology and postmortem sectioning of cervical spines show that radiology misses the vast majority of the traumatic lesions (2,3).

The few published postmortem studies of cervical spinal injuries vary widely in the rigor with which they searched for injuries (1,2,20,21). Davis' (20) series of 50 cases, showed that disc injuries are more common than radiology suggests, but only serial sectioning reveals the full extent of the injuries (2,3,5). As the few published serial sectioning studies rely on small numbers of cases, there is a need for a more comprehensive autopsy study based on serial sectioning.

Neck sprain or "whiplash" injuries are associated with acute neck pain and referred pain. A 20-40% proportion of the injuries progresses to a chronic pain syndrome (22,23,24). The diagnosis of the neck pathology associated with the injury is severely hampered by the inability of current imaging modalities to demonstrate the lesions which may be present or by the prohibitive expense of applying magnetic resonance imaging to all the acute injuries, without any reliable way of predicting which injuries will go on to a chronic pain state.

It is important to distinguish the lesions of injury from those of aging. The repeated translation and shearing which accompany normal movements, produce uncovertebral clefts in late childhood and transverse fissures in young adult discs. These extend from the uncovertebral clefts, across the posterior half of each cervical disc, midway between the vertebral end plates (25,26). Trauma to the disc, on the other hand, usually tears the cervical disc at its junction with the vertebral end plate (3).

MATERIALS AND METHODS

In a study of 180 sagittally sectioned cervical spines from subjects of all ages, 109 were from blunt trauma fatalities. The spines were carefully removed at autopsy, together with the base of the skull, to include the complete atlanto-occipital joints and lateral and antero-posterior x-rays were taken of the specimens. They were fixed by immersion in 10% formalin for 10 days, embedded in 6% gelatin, frozen at $-70°C$ on dry ice for 48 hours and sectioned in 2.5 mm slices on a band saw with a specially made guide to ensure regular and predictable section thickness (5). The sections were carefully washed and examined with the naked eye and using an M3 dissecting microscope. Forty of the injured spines were sectioned with the cord in situ. In the remaining 63 injured spines, the cord was removed for separate examination after a laminectomy which was carefully done to avoid any damage to the zygapophyseal joints.

The cervical spines sectioned were from 74 male and 35 female fatal injuries. The age distribution of the blunt trauma fatalities is shown in Figure 1. The age-related prevalence peaked in the 20-29 decade. The causes of death were, in order of frequency, head injuries, chest injuries, multiple injuries [usually to chest and head], spinal injuries and sequelae of injury such as stroke, heart failure or pneumonia. Motor vehicle trauma accounted for 72 of the fatalities [50 vehicle occupants; 22 motorcyclists, cyclists or pedestrians], falls and blows to the head for 34, and sporting injuries for the remaining three.

Each section was examined and photographed using a Pentax camera with a macro lens and a Leitz M3 dissecting microscope with camera attached. The position and nature of all visible lesions were marked on a standard diagram of the cervical spine and the data entered on a spread sheet and analyzed according to the segment injured and the nature of the injury. Data from the general autopsy and a brief account of the accident by a police officer attending the scene, were used to classify the probable injury mechanisms.

FIGURE 1. Age distribution of injuries: The number of fatal injuries per decade for the 109 spines. Three quarters of the injuries occur in the 10-50 age range, peaking in the third decade.

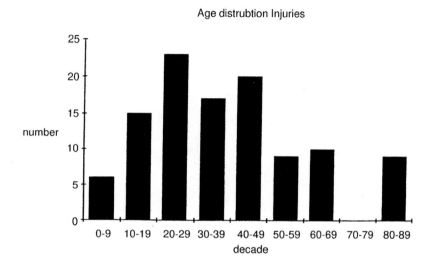

Age distrubtion Injuries

RESULTS

Out of the 109 fatal injuries, traumatic lesions were found in 102 cervical spines [94%]; similar lesions were not found in the spines from the non-traumatic fatalities. The spinal injury severity varied from a minor tear in a disc, or bleeding into a facet joint, to fractures or dislocations with cord laceration. Most injuries involved the joints rather than the vertebrae; e.g., injuries to the discs were four times more frequent than fractures to the vertebrae. Including all injuries, disc and facet injuries were almost equally common, though disc injuries were more common in the upper segments and facet injuries were more frequent at C6-7 [Figure 2]. The disc and facet injuries were classified as severe or minor and also according to the motion segment involved [Figures 3 and 4].

Postmortem radiology. A study of 58 sets of postmortem x-rays judged to be of acceptable diagnostic quality, compared to the study of the sectioned specimens as a standard, failed to detect 199 [64.4%] of the 309 lesions visible in the sections; 93.5% of the minor lesions [mainly rim lesions and facet hemarthroses] were missed by the radiologist who also made 32 false positive diagnoses of traumatic lesions.

FIGURE 2. Disc and facet injuries: Overall, there are about equal numbers of disc and facet injuries, with a slight excess of disc injuries at higher levels and more facet injuries at C6-7.

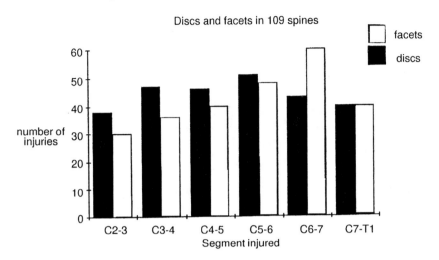

FIGURE 3. Disc trauma: The distribution of severe and minor injuries is shown. Severe injuries are disc avulsions, disruptions and traumatic herniations; they peak at C5-6 and C6-7. Minor injuries include rim lesions and bleeding into the disc; these peak at C3-4 and C4-5.

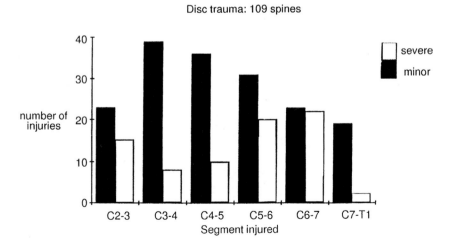

FIGURE 4. Facet trauma: Minor injuries include hemarthroses, capsular and articular cartilage damage; Severe injuries are fractures and dislocations. Both minor and severe injuries peak at C5-6 and C6-7.

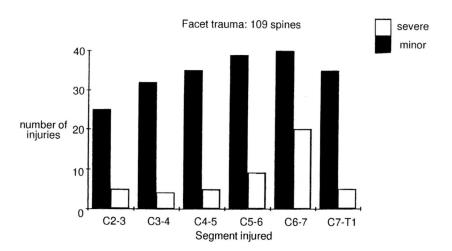

Forces and mechanisms of injury. In the 102 cases which showed neck injury, the recorded nature and position of injuries to the head, brain torso and viscera, suggested that the neck injury was secondary to head impact in 54 cases, that the neck injury was due to primary acceleration of the torso, without head injury, in 37 cases and that the neck injury was secondary to a combination of head and torso injuries in 11 cases. Fifty injuries were from high velocity impacts [>60 kph], mostly motor vehicle trauma [MVT]; 52 spines were injured at impact speeds judged to be less than 60 kph [Table 1]. Ten of these injuries were in vehicle occupants in city traffic crashes; 7 of them were not wearing seat belts and 3 had head impacts despite wearing seat belts. Some impact fatalities were in cyclists or pedestrians hit by motor vehicles in city traffic; 32 of the under 60 kph impact injuries were due to falls or blows to the head.

From the nature of the spinal lesions, the evidence of other injuries and the police reports of the accident, the major force vector producing the injuries was deduced. On this basis, 54% were classified as extension or extension compression injuries, 15% as axial compression injuries and 27% as flexion or lateral flexion injuries; 4% of the injuries could not be classified. Most extension, extension compression or axial compression injuries were from cranio-facial impacts. In these cases, the spines showed

TABLE 1. Injury Types by Estimated Impact Speed.

Type of Injury	>60 km/h	<60 km/h
Fracture or dislocation	24	15
Severe injury, normal alignment	18	12
Minor injury	8	25
Total	**50**	**52**

anterior distraction injuries, including anterior rim lesions or disc avulsions with anterior longitudinal ligament strains or tears, and posterior compression injuries, with posterior disc contusions, facet hemarthroses, or fractures to the facet tips or to an articular pillar. Where there was posterior longitudinal ligament damage or ligamentum flavum rupture, the injury was classified as a flexion injury.

Upper cervical injuries. There were 19 atlanto-occipital or atlanto-axial dislocations and more numerous less severe injuries to the capsule or synovial folds of these joints. The most common injury was bruising of the synovial folds in the atlanto-axial joints, found in 59 spines, most often involving the posterior synovial folds, and often associated with a hematoma around the C2 nerve, behind the C1-2 lateral joint [Figure 5]. There were 15 fractures of C1 and 17 fractures of C2, nine of the latter involving the dens. Upper cervical injuries were described in detail in a previous publication (27).

Spinal cord and nerve injury. Injuries to the spinal cord or brain stem were found in 25% of the 109 fatalities and 22% of the MV occupants. Nerve root injuries [Figure 6] were seen in 44 dorsal root ganglia [DRG] in 14% of the 109 spines and in 34.5% of the subgroup of 29 who survived the injury for between two hours and seven days. The DRG most frequently injured were C5 and C8 [eight each], then C3 and C7 [seven each]. The most common injury mechanisms for DRG injury were extension or side-bending. The DRG injuries were often present, without accompanying musculoskeletal injury or with only minor disc or facet injury at the same level. Vertebral artery injuries were infrequent, except in severe, complete dislocations, but bleeding from injured vertebral veins was common. The arterial injuries were mostly dissections of the intima and media, with intravascular thrombosis.

Fractures. These [excluding facet fractures, classified as joint injuries] were classified as:

- *minor* fractures–tear drop avulsion fractures of a corner of the vertebral body or small compression fractures of the vertebral body end plate;
- *severe* fractures–vertebral body wedging, burst fracture, or fracture through a lamina, pedicle or spinous process. The C2 vertebra was the one most often fractured, in 17 cases; nine of these were dens fractures. The next most common fracture site was C6, in 16 cases, where nine wedge or burst fractures were seen in axial compression injuries.

Disc injuries. These were again classified as severe and minor injuries. The minor injuries include small, localized, transverse tears of the annulus fibrosus at the vertebral rim [rim lesions] or bleeding into the disc, without disc disruption [Figure 7]. These were most common at C3-4 and C4-5 [Figure 3]. The severe disc injuries include complete or partial avulsion of the disc [Figure 8] from the vertebra, often through the cartilage plate [in younger subjects], traumatic disruption of the disc [in older subjects] and

FIGURE 5. C1-2 soft tissue injury: A sagittal section of the right lateral atlanto-axial joint of a 66 year old male driver whose car swerved off the road and hit a tree resulting in fatal head and thoracic injuries. He had a stiff lower cervical spine and suffered upper cervical injuries including a hematoma in the posterior inta-articular synovial fold [S], extending backwards around the C2 dorsal root ganglion [G].

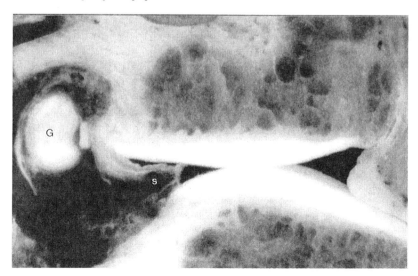

FIGURE 6. Nerve root injury: Central interstitial hemorrhage into the C3 dorsal root ganglion [G] in a 49 year old man, who tripped and fell backwards, striking his head on a concrete floor with fracture of the skull base and subsequent cerebral edema. The ganglion lies in the space between the C2-3 facet joint [Z] and the vertebral artery [VA].

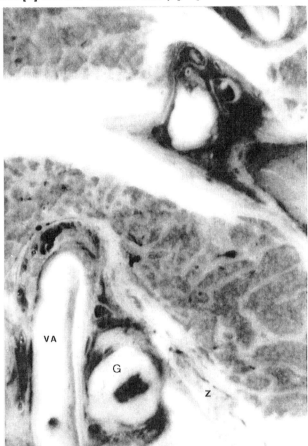

traumatic herniations of part of the disc into the spinal canal [Figure 9]. Severe disc injuries were most frequently seen at C5-6 and C6-7.

In discs with rim lesions the longitudinal ligaments were intact [Figure 7] and in many disc avulsions, the longitudinal ligaments were either strained or only partly torn. Even when the anterior longitudinal ligament [ALL] was ruptured, the small anterior muscles were not usually torn, showing only intramuscular hemorrhage [Figure 8]. Of 87 individuals with disc

FIGURE 7. Rim lesions: Midline sagittal sections of the C4-5 and C5-6 discs from a 41 year old man show linear tears in the anterior annulus [arrowed] near the vertebral rim, with bleeding into the tears and spread of blood between the annular lamellae. The lower disc also shows bleeding into the posterior annulus fibrosus. The anterior longitudinal ligament is intact. This passenger was thrown out of an off-road vehicle travelling at 30-40 kph, onto sand, and died of a subarachnoid hemorrhage.

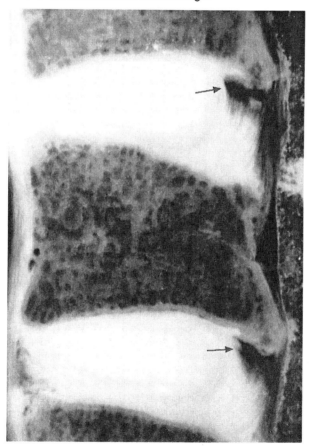

injuries, 33 showed damage to one or both longitudinal ligaments; 27 showed ALL damage, eight with complete tears and 19 with partial tears or strains; 17 showed posterior longitudinal ligament damage, five with complete tears and 12 with partial tears or strains.

Facet injuries. Minor injuries include hemarthroses, capsular tears or

FIGURE 8. Disc avulsion: A sagittal section of the C6-7 disc from a 20 year old man who died of head injuries when thrown from a fork lift truck as it rolled on its side when doing a fast U-turn. The disc is avulsed along the cartilage plate. The anterior longitudinal ligament is torn and the anterior muscle [M] is bruised, but not torn. Severe disc injuries in younger subjects are usually avulsions at the disc vertebral junction.

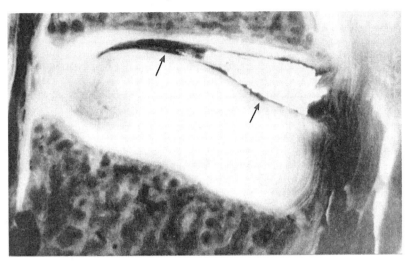

articular cartilage damage, severe injuries are facet fractures involving the joint cavity. The injury prevalence peaks at C5-6 and C6-7 for both types of injury [Figure 4]. Examples of hemarthroses, articular cartilage damage and fractures are shown in Figures 10-12.

Comparison of head impact and "whiplash." Comparing the spinal injuries in two groups: those with primary head injuries and those arising from primary torso injuries, with no significant head impact, the injuries were broadly similar in severity and distribution in the two groups.

DISCUSSION

Serial saggital sectioning of the spine reveals many more traumatic lesions than can be seen by postmortem radiology or by simple hemisection of the spine (2,3,5). Radiology misses the majority of the disc lesions, all the facet joint hemarthroses and many facet fractures, while hemisection does not display the facet joints. In a postmortem radiological study, Alker (28) found cervical spinal injuries in 21% of 146 fatal injuries. Our

FIGURE 9. Disc herniation: A sagittal section of the C6-7 disc from a 52 year old woman thrown out of the rear seat of a 4 wheel drive vehicle which rolled over at speed on a gravel road. Death was from head injuries. The injured disc shows a large posterior disc herniation [H] indenting the anterior cord, and a small anterior rim lesion [arrowed].

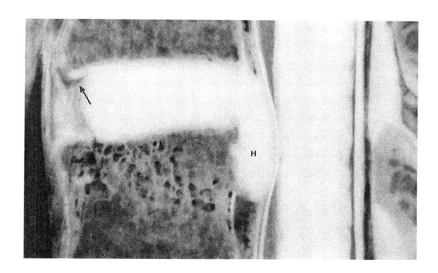

study demonstrated injuries in 94% of 109 fatal injuries. The lesions are consistent in appearance, with bleeding into the lesions; they are absent in non-traumatic fatalities, in this study and a previous study using a different sectioning method (3).

Relevance to "whiplash." The relevance of these autopsy observations, mostly in severe high velocity trauma, to clinical cervical spine injuries requires careful consideration. The mechanism of injury differs in one major respect. Classical "whiplash" is a non-impact injury but a large proportion of the cervical spinal injuries in this study are secondary to head impact. However, a comparison of the nature and distribution of the cervical spinal injuries in those subjects with primary head impact and those without head injury but with primary acceleration of the torso, fails to reveal any significant differences in the nature and distribution of injuries.

Injury severity and force or velocity of impact. The average force producing injury in this autopsy series is greater than for most whiplash, but there is a very wide range from simple falls at ground level, and head blows in fist fights, to high velocity car smashes. Comparing the spinal

FIGURE 10. Hemarthroses: The sagittally sectioned facet joints of this 52 year old woman [the same subject as in Figure 5] show hemarthroses [H], with capsular and posterior muscle damage [M].

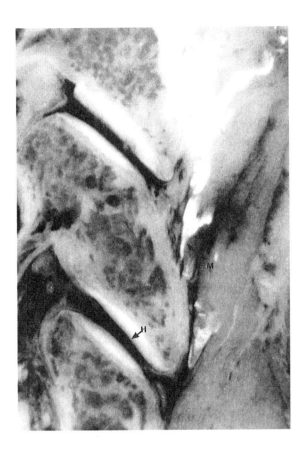

injuries in those with greater or less than 60 kph impacts, there are more severe injuries and a greater number of injuries per spine in the high velocity smashes than in the under 60 kph impacts, but some spinal injuries in the under 60 kph group are severe [Table 1]. The severity of the neck injury did not correlate well with the severity of the head injury or chest injury causing death. The spinal injury severity ranged from zero, seven spines showing no injury, to spinal injury causing death. Comparing the severity of neck injury in this series, with the fracture dislocations with

FIGURE 11. Articular cartilage damage: The C7-T1 joint from a 57 year old woman, a seat-belted, rear seat passenger in a car which struck a tree at 90kph. Death resulted from multiple rib fractures with lung damage and intra-thoracic hemorrhage. The articular cartilage shows partial detachment [D] and bruising, with hemarthrosis in the joint. There is traumatic detachment of the posterior muscle insertion into the lamina below [arrows].

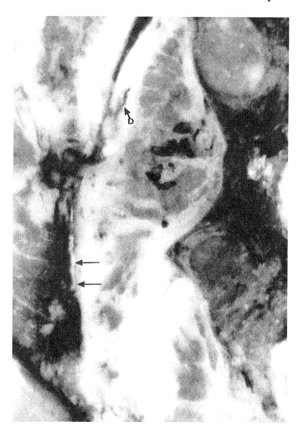

SCI in patients admitted to spinal units, the average spinal injury severity is less in this autopsy series than in the spinal cord injured patients. In this series only 25% showed SCI; about two thirds showed one or more severe segmental injuries and one third showed only minor injuries. In many cases in this series, the forces producing the spinal injuries are comparable

FIGURE 12. Facet tip fracture: The sagittally sectioned C6-7 zygapophyseal joint from a 16 year old male struck on the head with a club showing fracture of the tip of the C7 superior articular process [SAP]. Parts of the fragmented facet tip lie anterior to the SAP. There are hemarthroses in the C6-7 and C7-T1 joints.

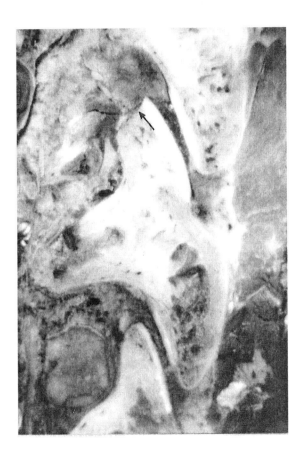

to the forces causing spinal injury in survivors of road trauma. Fatal spinal injury can occur in a relatively minor incident, like a fall at ground level, in elderly subjects with stiff lower cervical spines (29).

Diagnosis of pathology in survivors of neck injury. Routine radiological investigation frequently fails to demonstrate lesions in a painful neck, it is impractical to do MRI in all neck injuries and if MRI is used the radiologist needs to be able to distinguish age changes from traumatic lesions. Severe injuries are often present in a normally aligned spine [Table 1]. Lesions similar to the acute injuries demonstrated in this study are likely to occur in a proportion of survivors of car accidents with neck pain, but most of these lesions will not be demonstrable by x-rays in living patients. Rim lesions have been found at autopsy in a group of survivors with chronic neck pain, who died of other causes one to four years after a neck injury, and also, in the form of vacuum clefts in radiographs, in a group of patients with chronic neck pain (30). The consistency of the injury patterns observed in this cadaver study suggests that if the forces are severe enough, similar injuries will usually be produced.

Relevance to acute neck pain. The injuries most frequently seen, are tears of the outer annulus fibrosus and trauma to the capsules of facet joints. The outer annulus and the fibrous capsules of facet joints are well innervated and would be likely to be painful when injured in survivors of neck trauma (31,32,33,34,35). It is important for clinicians and radiologists to be aware of the possibility that such lesions may be present after trauma.

Possible relevance to chronic neck pain. It is often asserted that "soft tissue" or ligamentous injuries heal rapidly. On the other hand, injuries to avascular cartilages like intervertebral discs or articular cartilage heal slowly and leave "degenerative" sequelae. Experimental and Imaging observations confirm that tears in discs persist unhealed for six to 18 months and are associated with degenerative changes (3,11,36). Similarly, articular cartilage surface lacerations apparently lack the ability to heal, while deep lesions fill with vascular fibrous tissue (37).

Chronic pain syndromes often result from neck injuries, especially after motor vehicle accidents and the signs and symptoms are remarkably similar in different countries (9,22,23,24). In the absence of a generally applicable imaging technique capable of demonstrating the trauma lesions, an awareness of their possible nature enables clinicians to target them with suitable investigations (12,30,38). Careful and skillful clinical examination of the discs and facets is mandatory when pain persists after injury (39) and the relevance of pain provocation and elimination techniques in diagnosis is obvious (9,30). In a study of 50 consecutive "whiplash" patients with chronic pain, Barnsley et al. (38) demonstrated by pain provocation and elimination tests that the pain arose from the zygapophyseal joints in 54% of the patients. In the absence of adequate investigation, symptoms may be inadvertently attributed to psycho-social factors, when in fact there may be persisting, undiagnosed peripheral nociception (9,40,41). Appropriate investigation can often provide the accurate segmental diagnosis of a pain source which is essential for effective treatment of neck pain (30).

REFERENCES

1. Cain CMJ, Ryan GA, Fraser R, Potter G, et al.: Cervical spine injuries in road traffic crashes in South Australia. Aust NZ J Surg 59: 15-19, 1989.

2. Jonsson H, Bring G, Rauschning W, et al.: Hidden cervical injuries in traffic accident victims with skull fractures. J Spinal Disorders 4(3): 251-263, 1991.

3. Taylor JR, Twomey LT: Acute Injuries to cervical joints. Spine 18: 1115-1122, 1993.

4. MacNab I: The whiplash syndrome. Clin Neurosurg 20: 232-24, 1973.

5. Kakulas BA, Taylor JR: Pathology of injuries of the vertebral column and spinal cord. In Handbook of Clinical Neurology: Spinal Cord Trauma, ed. Bruyn GW, Vinken PJ, Klawans HL, Frankel HL: 61: 21-51. Amsterdam Elsevier Science Publishers, 1992.

6. Holdsworth FW: Fractures, dislocations and fracture-dislocations of the spine. J Bone & Joint Surg 52A: 1534-1551, 1963.

7. Huelke DF, Nuscholz GS: Cervical spine biomechanics. J Orthopaedic Research 4: 232-245, 1986.

8. Pal GP, Sherk HH: The vertical stability of the cervical spine. Spine 13: 447-449, 1988.

9. Barnsley L, Lord S, Bogduk N: Whiplash injury. Pain 58: 283-307, 1994.

10. Bedbrook GM: Spinal injuries with tetraplegia and paraplegia. J Bone Joint Surg 61B: 267-283, 1979.

11. Davis SJ, Teresi LM, Bradley WG, Ziemba MA, Bloze AE: Cervical spine hyperextension injuries: MR findings. Radiology 180: 245-25, 1991.

12. Jonsson H, Cesarini K, Sahlstedt B, Rauschning W: Findings and outcome in whiplash-type neck distortions. Spine 19:2733-2743, 1994.

13. Dalinka MK, Kessler H, Weiss M: The radiographic evaluation of spinal trauma. Emerg Med Clin of Nth Am. 3: 475-490, 1985.

14. Edeiken-Monroe B, Wagner LK, Harris JH: Hyperextension dislocation of the cervical spine. AJR 146: 803-808, 1986.

15. Harris JH, Edeiken-Monroe B, Kopaniky DR: A practical classification of acute cervical spine injuries. Orthop Clin of Nth Am 17: 15-30, 1986.

16. Gerrelts BD, Petersen EU, Marby J, Petersen SR: Delayed diagnosis of cervical spine injuries. J Trauma 31(12): 1622-1626, 1991.

17. Woodring JH, Lee C: Limitations of cervical radiography in the evaluation of acute cervical trauma. J Trauma 34: 32-39, 1993.

18. Cintron E, Gilula LA, Murphy WA, Gehweiler JA: The widened disc space: A sign of cervical hyperextension injury. Radiology 141: 639-644, 1981.

19. Daffner RH, Deeb ZL, Rothfus WE: Fingerprints of vertebral trauma: a unifying concept based on mechanisms. Skeletal Radiol 15: 518-525, 1986.

20. Davis D, Bohlman H, Walker AE, Fisher R, Robinson R: The pathological findings in fatal craniospinal injuries. J Neurosurg 34: 603-613, 1971.

21. Aufdermaur M: Spinal injuries in juveniles: Necropsy findings in twelve cases. J Bone Joint Surg 56B : 513-519, 1974.

22. Deans GT, Magaillard JN, Kerr M, Rutherford WH: Neck sprains: a major cause of disability following car accidents. Injury 18: 10-12, 1987.

23. Porter KM: Neck sprains after car accidents: a common cause of long term disability. BMJ editorial, 298: 973-974, 1989.

24. Gargan MF, Bannister GC: Long term prognosis of soft tissue injuries of the neck. J Bone Joint Surg 72B: 901-903, 1990.

25. Tondury G: Anatomie fonctionelle des petites articulations du rachis. Annales de Medecine Physique XV: 173-19, 1972.

26. Taylor JR, Twomey LT: Functional and Applied Anatomy of the Cervical Spine. In Physical Therapy of the Cervical and Thoracic Spine, ed Grant R: 1-25. Edinburgh, New York, Churchill Livingstone, 1994.

27. Schönström N, Twomey L, Taylor J: The lateral atlanto-axial joints and their synovial folds: an in vitro study of soft tissue injuries and fractures. J Trauma 35: 886-892, 1993.

28. Alker GJ, Young S, Leslie EV, et al.: Postmortem radiology of head and neck injuries in fatal traffic accidents. Radiology 114: 611-617, 1975.

29. Scher AT: Hyperextension trauma in the elderly: An easily overlooked spinal injury. J Trauma 23: 1066-1068, 1983.

30. Taylor JR, Finch P: Acute injury of the neck: anatomical and pathological basis of pain. Annals Academy of Medicine (Singapore) 22: 187-192, 1993.

31. Cloward RB: Cervical discography: A contribution to the etiology and mechanism of neck, shoulder, arm pain. Ann Surg 150: 1052-1064, 1959.

32. Bogduk N: The clinical anatomy of the cervical dorsal rami. Spine 7: 319-330, 1982.

33. Bogduk N: The innervation of cervical intervertebral discs. Spine 13: 2-8, 1987.

34. Mendel T, Wink CS, Zimny ML: Neural elements in human cervical intervertebral discs. Spine 17: 132-135, 1992.

35. Dwyer A, Aprill C, Bogduk N: Cervical zygapophyseal joint pain patterns. Spine 15: 453-457, 1990.

36. Osti OL, Vernon-Roberts B, Fraser RD: Annulus tears and intervertebral disc degeneration: an experimental study using an animal model. Spine 15: 762-767, 1990.

37. Mankin HJ: Current Concepts Review: The response of articular cartilage to mechanical injury. J Bone Joint Surgery 64A: 460-466, 1982.

38. Barnsley L, Lord S, Wallis B, Bogduk N: The prevalence of chronic cervical zygapophysial joint pain after whiplash. Spine, 20: 20-26, 1995.

39. Jull G, Bogduk N, Marsland A: The accuracy of manual diagnosis for cervical zygapophyseal joint pain syndromes. Med J Australia 148: 233-236, 1988.

40. Mersky H. Neck injury and the mind. Lancet editorial, 338:728-729, 1991.

41. Radanov BP, Dvorak J, Valach L: Cognitive deficits in patients after soft tissue injury of the cervical spine. Spine 17: 127-131, 1992.

The Cervical Synovial Joints
as Sources of Post-Traumatic Headache

Susan M. Lord
Nikolai Bogduk

SUMMARY. Objectives: To describe recent research which elucidates the role of the cervical synovial joints as sources of pain in patients with post-traumatic headache.

Findings: Recent research has demonstrated that the cervical synovial joints are innervated and that they can be potent sources of neck pain and headache if stimulated in normal subjects or if injured in patients. Postmortem studies of injured joints have revealed chondral and subchondral fractures, bruising/damage of the intra-articular inclusions, hemarthroses and capsular tears or avulsions. These acute lesions constitute the substrate for the development of post-traumatic arthritis and, consequently, chronic post-traumatic headache. Such lesions evade detection by conventional diagnostic tech-

Susan M. Lord, BMedSc, BMed[Hons], is Research Fellow, Cervical Spine Research Unit, The University of Newcastle, Australia. Nikolai Bogduk, BSc[Med], MB BS, MD, PhD, FAFRM[RACP], is Professor of Anatomy and Director of the Cervical Spine Research Unit, The University of Newcastle, Australia.

Address correspondence to: Dr. Susan M. Lord, Cervical Spine Research Unit, Faculty of Medicine, The University of Newcastle, Callaghan, NSW 2308, Australia.

This study was supported by a grant from the Motor Accidents Authority of New South Wales. All procedures were performed at the Newcastle Mater Misericordiae Hospital, Waratah, New South Wales, Australia.

[Haworth co-indexing entry note]: "The Cervical Synovial Joints as Sources of Post-Traumatic Headache." Lord, Susan M., and Nikolai Bogduk. Co-published simultaneously in *Journal of Musculoskeletal Pain* [The Haworth Medical Press, an imprint of The Haworth Press, Inc.] Vol. 4, No. 4, 1996, pp. 81-94; and: *Musculoskeletal Pain Emanating from the Head and Neck: Current Concepts in Diagnosis, Management and Cost Containment* [ed: Murray E. Allen] The Haworth Medical Press, an imprint of The Haworth Press, Inc., 1996, pp. 81-94. Single or multiple copies of this article are available from The Haworth Document Delivery Service [1-800-342-9678, 9:00 a.m. - 5:00 p.m. [EST]. E-mail address: getinfo@haworth.com].

niques. However, the advent of innovative diagnostic approaches, including manipulative assessment, biomechanical analysis and controlled diagnostic injection techniques, has allowed the identification of painful cervical synovial joints *in vivo*. Using these diagnostic techniques, epidemiological studies have shown that the cervical zygapophysial joints [in particular C2-3] are common sources of post-traumatic headache.

Conclusions: These findings support the hypothesis that cervical synovial joint pain is a real and common clinical entity. Controlled diagnostic blocks are the only reliable means whereby this condition can be identified. Controlled blocks provide a criterion standard against which other diagnostic techniques could be calibrated in the future. *[Article copies available from The Haworth Document Delivery Service: 1-800-342-9678. E-mail address: getinfo@haworth.com]*

KEYWORDS. Cervical synovial joint, headache, trauma, whiplash

INTRODUCTION

The cervical synovial joints include the atlanto-occipital joints, the median and lateral atlanto-axial joints and the zygapophysial joints found along the posterior cervical vertebral column at intervertebral levels C2-3 to C7-T1. As possible sources of headache their role has, in the past, been only conjectural. Extrapolation from experience with synovial joints elsewhere in the body predicts that the cervical synovial joints could be affected by pathological processes which cause pain, including inflammation, infection and trauma. Of these afflictions, trauma is perhaps the most common and yet it is the most controversial.

That major fractures and dislocations can affect the upper cervical synovial joints is not disputed. Such lesions are usually suggested by the clinical presentation and can be confirmed using conventional imaging investigations. In this setting, clinicians have little trouble in ascribing the presence of neck pain and headache to the damaged structures.

However, far more common, and certainly more controversial, is the patient who presents with post-traumatic headache (1), but who has normal neurological examination and normal x-rays.

Pathology

A number of different research approaches has been employed to demonstrate the range of lesions which might befall the cervical synovial joints as a result of trauma.

In studies in which experimental animals or cadavers have been subjected to whiplash motion, injuries to the cervical zygapophysial joints are amongst the most common and most consistent lesion produced. The lesions include impaction fractures, tears of the joint capsules and damage to the articular cartilage.

Post-mortem studies of victims of motor vehicle accidents reveal that cervical synovial joint injuries are common (2), being present in 86% of necks examined in one study (3). The lesions include fractures involving either the supporting articular pillars or the articular surfaces themselves, capsular tears and avulsions, rupture, displacement or hematomas of the intraarticular meniscoids, hemarthroses and damage or fissuring of the articular cartilage.

Even for small fractures of synovial joints, plain radiography is extremely insensitive. In one study in which some 73 lesions of zygapophysial joints were identified at post-mortem, only four were evident on plain films of the specimens, even retrospectively (3). Nevertheless, fractures and dislocations of the cervical synovial joints have been identified in patients suffering from cervical trauma, when special imaging techniques have been used (4-10). However, there have been no systematic studies of patients with post-traumatic headache using special imaging techniques so, the prevalence of small articular fractures is not known, and may be under-appreciated. It is here proposed that diagnostic blocks may prove that a particular joint is symptomatic even though no lesion is evident.

Innervation

The cervical zygapophysial joints are innervated by articular branches which arise from the medial branches of the cervical dorsal rami [Figure 1, 2] (11,12). The C2-3 zygapophysial joint is innervated by the superficial medial branch of the C3 dorsal ramus which is large and is known as the third occipital nerve (13). Beyond the C2-3 zygapophysial joint, the third occipital nerve furnishes muscle branches to the semispinalis capitis and becomes cutaneous over the suboccipital region. In this respect the C3 dorsal ramus is the only cervical dorsal ramus below C2 that regularly has a cutaneous distribution. The C3-4 to C7-T1 zygapophysial joints have a dual innervation derived from the deep medial branches of the cervical dorsal rami immediately above and below the joint. Beyond the zygapophysial joints the medial branches of the cervical dorsal rami supply the semispinalis and multifidus muscles. Those from C4 to C8 typically lack any cutaneous branches (13).

FIGURE 1. An illustration of a dorsal view of the atlanto-occipital and atlanto-axial articulations. The vertebral arches, tectorial membrane and posterior longitudinal and apical ligaments have been removed to demonstrate the innervation of the right upper cervical synovial joints. Articular branches innervating the atlanto-occipital [AO] and lateral atlanto-axial [AA] joints arise from the C1 and C2 ventral rami [VR] respectively. The median atlanto-axial joint and the transverse and alar ligaments are innervated by branches of the C1 to C3 sinuvertebral nerves [SVN].

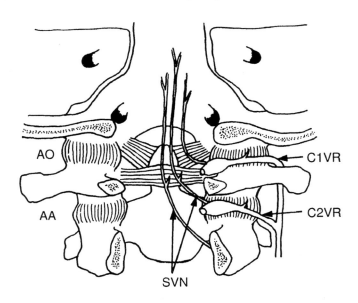

Pain

That somatic pain from cervical structures innervated by the C1-3 spinal nerves can be referred to the head has been established for some time (14-16). Nociceptive afferents from cervical structures synapse on second order neurons in the spinal nucleus of the trigeminal nerve [Figure 3]. Consequently, pain arising from the upper four cervical synovial joints would, theoretically, be perceived as pain in the neck and in the distribution of the relevant branches of the trigeminal nerve.

Experimental studies in normal volunteers have clearly shown that the cervical synovial joints can be a source of local pain and referred pain to the head. Distension of these joints with injections of contrast medium produces patterns of pain that are reasonably characteristic of the segment being stimulated (17-19) [Figure 4]. In particular, stimulation of the atlan-

FIGURE 2. An illustration of a dorso-lateral view of the left cervical dorsal rami in the plane of multifidus [deep to semispinalis capitis]. The lateral branches of the cervical dorsal rami have been cut at their origin. The third occipital nerve [ton] innervates the C2-3 zygapophysial joint, as it crosses the dorso-lateral aspect of the joint. Alternatively, the communicating branch [c] between C2 and C3 may innervate at C2-3 joint. Below C2-3, the deep medial branches [m] send articular branches [a] to the zygapophysial joints, and then end in multifidus [M]. The superficial medial branches pass deep or dorsal to semispinalis cervicis [SSCe] to become cutaneous. TP, transverse process of C1; SP, spinous process of T1; gon, greater occipital nerve.

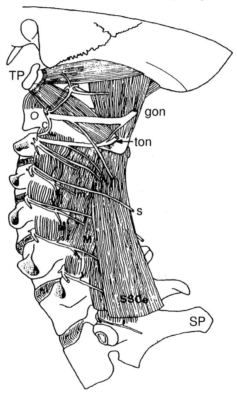

to-occipital joints, the lateral atlanto-axial joints and the C2-3 zygapophysial joints produced pain that was referred to various regions of the head.

Clinical studies have shown that certain patients with headache can be relieved of their pain by blocking cervical synovial joints with local anesthetic (19-36). Patients with painful atlanto-occipital and atlanto-axial

FIGURE 3. A posterior view of the brainstem illustrating the disposition of the nuclei of the trigeminal nerve [pr, principal nucleus; po, pars oralis; pi, pars interpolaris; pc, pars caudalis]. The pars caudalis is continuous with the spinal grey matter. This column of grey matter receives afferents from the spinal tract of trigeminal nerve [Sp tract] and from the C1 to C3 spinal nerves [shown on the left]. The inset on the right shows the relative distribution within the nucleus of afferents from the three divisions of the trigeminal nerve [V1, V2 and V3].

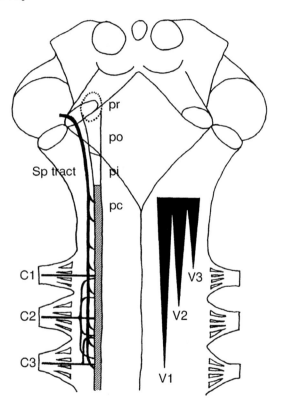

joints have had their pain relieved by intra-articular (29,32,37,38) or peri-articular (32) injections of local anesthetic. Patients with pain stemming from the cervical zygapophysial joints have had their headache relieved either by anesthetizing the joint with intra-articular injections of local anesthetic (20-22,24-28) or by blocking the medial branches of the dorsal rami that supply the painful joint (19,23,25,28).

FIGURE 4. Composite maps depicting the characteristic distribution of pain emanating from the atlanto-occipital [AO] and lateral atlanto-axial joints [AA] and C2-3 to C6-7 zygapophysial joints (17,18).

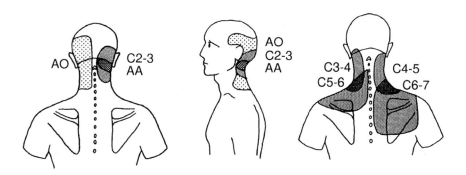

DIAGNOSIS

Conventional Diagnostic Algorithm

When neck pathology is suspected, apart from history and physical examination, it is appropriate to employ hematological, biochemical, immunological and/or imaging investigations in order to confirm or refute the clinical impression. However, the yield from this approach will be meager. Patterns of referred pain from the various upper cervical synovial joints are not mutually exclusive, the overlap is so great as to render their predictive value doubtful. Moreover, muscles, ligaments, dura and discs which share the same segmental innervation as the upper cervical synovial joints refer pain to similar locations (13,39-41).

The location of the axial synovial joints deep to multiple layers of posterior vertebral muscles renders them relatively inaccessible. Examination pressure applied to one cervical muscle or joint is transmitted to underlying and adjacent muscles and joints. Similarly, it is difficult to execute active and passive movements of an isolated joint without also influencing the contralateral and adjacent joints. False-positive diagnoses can arise because symptoms are often attributed to the presence of age-related changes on radiological examination, which can be asymptomatic (42-44). False-negative diagnoses occur when the diagnostic tool is insufficiently sensitive. Post-mortem studies have demonstrated pathology that was missed by plain radiography (3,45) and single photon emission computed tomography [SPECT] scans (46). This paucity of valid, conventional, diagnostic tools has necessitated exploration of non-conventional or novel approaches to the diagnosis of pain from the cervical synovial joints.

Manipulative Assessment

There have been many claims regarding the accuracy of manual diagnosis (47) but few data. Only one study compared manual diagnosis to the criterion standard of diagnostic local anesthetic blocks (48). The authors found the sensitivity and specificity of the manual examination technique to be 100%. The manual therapist correctly identified all patients with proven joint pain, the symptomatic and asymptomatic segments. The ability of other manual examiners to replicate these results has not been tested.

Controlled Diagnostic Injection Techniques

Controlled diagnostic anesthetic "block" injections may offer the only definitive means of identifying painful cervical synovial joints. If the patient's pain is completely relieved then the tested joint must have been the source of that pain. If unrelieved then the tested joint can be excluded.

In principle, a cervical synovial joint could be anesthetized by injection of local anesthetic either into the joint itself or onto the nerves supplying the joint. Historically, intra-articular blocks are more senior (49,50). Intra-articular blocks were thought to be anatomically specific and offered a therapeutic advantage; putatively therapeutic agents could be injected intra-articularly if the response to local anesthetic was positive (20-22,26,37,38).

However, intra-articular blocks are disadvantageous in that they are technically demanding and time consuming, and patients risk significant procedural pain, allergy to contrast medium and septic arthritis. In less experienced hands, patients might also risk technical misadventure with damage to neural or vascular tissue. Moreover, there is evidence that intra-articular blocks may not be as target-specific as had been assumed previously. Fluid injected intra-articularly can escape from a synovial joint via capsular deficiencies or tears (26,27,37,49), anesthetising adjacent structures and, thereby, rendering the block non-specific. However, this problem may be overcome by using small volumes of injectate together with fastidious radiographic monitoring of the dilution and spread of contrast medium.

Whereas the articular branches supplying the atlanto-occipital and atlanto-axial joints lie so close to the spinal nerves that a specific articular nerve block is impossible, the medial branches innervating the zygapophysial joints are accessible and geographically discrete. Hence, for the diagnosis of zygapophysial joint pain, the most expeditious approach is to block the medial branch[es] supplying the joint. In response to expressed concerns regarding non-specific spread of local anesthetic to adjacent nerves or muscles, the reliability of cervical medial branch blocks was examined. Anatomical and radiological studies demonstrated medial branch blocks to be valid and target-specific (13-51).

Irrespective of the technique employed, diagnostic blocks rely on the patient's self-report of relief. Therefore, blocks may be vulnerable to a number of confounding factors which might result in a high proportion of false-positive diagnoses. Relief may be reported for reasons other than the pharmacological effect of the local anesthetic administered. Expectancy and classical conditioning may result in placebo responses (52,53) or the patient's pain may be coincidentally relieved, for example, by taking the day off work or by lying in a certain position on the x-ray table. The false-positive rate of single, uncontrolled cervical zygapophysial joint blocks was found to be as high 27%.

Therefore, control blocks are mandatory. Although placebo controls such as normal saline are the reputed ideal they are difficult to implement on a routine clinical basis and might be considered unethical in some circumstances. A more pragmatic form of control can be the use of different local anesthetic agents on different occasions, a paradigm known as comparative local anesthetic blocks (54-56). In a single- or double-blind setting, two local anesthetics with different durations of pharmacological action [commonly lignocaine and bupivacaine] are administered in random order on two separate occasions. A positive diagnosis is made if the patient exhibits reproducible, complete relief and correctly identifies the longer-acting agent (34).

EPIDEMIOLOGY

The prevalence of painful atlanto-occipital and median and lateral atlanto-axial joints amongst patients with post-traumatic headache is currently unknown. Although there seems to be consensus amongst practitioners of musculoskeletal medicine that these conditions are common, few case reports have appeared in the scientific literature (29,32,37), let alone prospective cohort studies.

On the other hand, much is known about the prevalence of cervical zygapophysial joint pain (25,28,35,36). Although much of the focus has been on their ability to produce chronic neck pain, one recent paper specifically addressed the prevalence of cervical zygapophysial joint pain amongst patients with chronic post-traumatic headache [more than three months' duration] following whiplash injury (36). A series of 71 consecutive patients with post-traumatic headache was studied using randomized, double-blind, comparative local anesthetic blocks. Of the 55 patients who completed investigation, 27 had their headache relieved by blocks of the C2-3 zygapophysial joint. This constitutes a prevalence of 49% with a 95% confidence interval of 36% to 62%. The prevalence of headache referred from lower cervical zygapophysial joints was smaller but not insignificant. Seven percent had headache from C3-4, 4% from C4-5, 13% from C5-6 and 2% had headache that was relieved by blocks of the C6-7 zygapophysial joint.

A stark difference in the relative prevalence of upper and lower cervical zygapophysial joint pain was observed depending on whether the dominant presenting complaint was headache or neck pain. Amongst patients with dominant headache, pain from the C2-3 zygapophysial joint accounted for more than half of cases. Pain from the C3-4 zygapophysial joint accounted for a small proportion of the remainder but joints below C3-4 were not implicated [Figure 5]. It may be that the atlanto-occipital or

FIGURE 5. Bar graph showing the prevalence of cervical zygapophysial joint [ZJ] pain amongst patients with post-traumatic headache following whiplash injury. The bar on the left shows the prevalence amongst patients whose dominant symptom was headache. That on the right shows the prevalence amongst patients for whom neck pain was the dominant complaint and headache was a secondary concern.

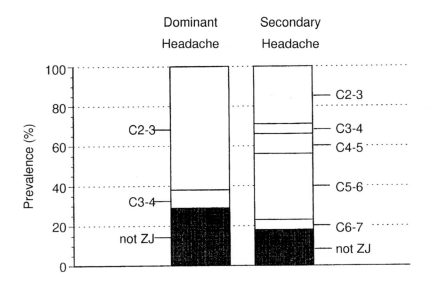

atlanto-axial joints are the source of pain in the other 29% but this hypothesis remains to be explored.

Amongst patients with dominant neck pain, for whom headache was a secondary complaint, C2-3 and C5-6 zygapophysial joint pain are almost equally common, each accounting for approximately 30% of cases. Headache referred from the other zygapophysial joints was recognized but was less common [Figure 5]. The mechanism whereby joints below C3-4 refer pain to the head is unknown. Referral via the trigeminocervical nucleus is unlikely since the trigeminal nucleus extends down only as far as the C3 segment (15). One hypothesis is that lower cervical zygapophysial joint pain causes reflex spasm of cervical muscles innervated by the C1-3 spinal segments. These muscles may become painful due to ischemia or due to failure at the myotendinous junctions or entheses.

In the epidemiology of post-traumatic headache there are many unknowns–the prevalence of pain from discs, dura and muscles. However, there is now a substantial body of anatomical, pathological and clinical evidence implicating the cervical synovial joints as the most common source of chronic headache after trauma. This evidence can no longer be ignored.

REFERENCES

1. Classification of Chronic Pain–Descriptions of Chronic Pain Syndromes and Definitions of Pain Terms. 2nd Ed. IASP Press, Seattle, 1994.

2. Bucholz RW, Burkhead WZ, Graham W, Petty C: Occult cervical spine injuries in fatal traffic accidents. J Trauma 119: 768-771, 1979.

3. Jónsson H,Jr., Bring G, Rauschning W, Sahlstedt B: Hidden cervical spine injuries in traffic accident victims with skull fractures. J Spinal Disorders 4: 251-263, 1991.

4. Abel MS: The radiology of chronic neck pain: sequelae of occult traumatic lesions. CRC Crit Rev Diag Imag 20: 27-78, 1982.

5. Binet EF, Moro JJ, Marangola JP, Hodge CJ: Cervical spine tomography in trauma. Spine 2: 163-172, 1977.

6. Smith GR, Beckly DE, Abel MS: Articular mass fracture: a neglected cause of post traumatic neck pain? Clin Radiol 27: 335-340, 1976.

7. Woodring JH, Goldstein SJ: Fractures of the articular processes of the cervical spine. Am J Roentgen 139: 341-344, 1982.

8. Abel MS: Occult traumatic lesions of the cervical vertebrae. CRC Crit Rev Clin Radiol Nucl Med 6: 469-553, 1975.

9. Jeffreys E: Soft tissue injuries, Disorders of the Cervical Spine. 2nd Ed. Butterworth-Heinemann, Oxford, 1993, pp. 105-112.

10. Clark CR, Igram CM, el Khoury GY, Ehara S: Radiographic evaluation of cervical spine injuries. Spine 13: 742-747, 1988.

11. Lazorthes G, Gaubert J: L'innervation des articulations inter-apophysaire vertebrales. Comptes Rendues de l'Association des Anatomistes,43 Reunion 488, 1956.

12. Kimmel DL: Innervation of spinal dura mater and dura mater of the posterior cranial fossa. Neurology 10: 800-809, 1961.

13. Bogduk N: The clinical anatomy of the cervical dorsal rami. Spine 7: 319-330, 1982.

14. Kerr FWL: A mechanism to account for frontal headache in cases of posterior fossa tumours. J Neurosurg 18: 605-609, 1961.

15. Kerr FWL: Trigeminal and cervical volleys. Arch Neurol 5: 171-178, 1961.

16. Kerr FWL: Structural relations of the spinal tract of the trigeminal nerve to the upper cervical roots and the solitary nucleus in the cat. Exp Neurol 4: 134-148, 1961.

17. Dreyfuss P, Michaelsen M, Fletcher D: Atlanto-occipital and lateral atlanto-axial joint pain patterns. Spine 19: 1125-1131, 1994.

18. Dwyer A, Aprill C, Bogduk N: Cervical zygapophyseal joint pain patterns. I: a study in normal volunteers. Spine 15: 453-457, 1990.

19. Aprill C, Dwyer A, Bogduk N: Cervical zygapophyseal joint pain patterns. II: a clinical evaluation. Spine 15: 458-461, 1990.

20. Dory MA: Arthrography of the cervical facet joints. Radiology 148: 379-382, 1983.

21. Wedel DJ, Wilson PR: Cervical facet arthrography. Regional Anesth 10: 7-11, 1985.

22. Dussault RG, Nicolet VM: Cervical facet joint arthrography. J Can Assoc Radiol 36: 79-80, 1985.

23. Bogduk N, Marsland A: On the concept of third occipital headache. J Neurol Neurosurg Psychiatry 49: 775-780, 1986.

24. Roy DF, Fleury J, Fontaine SB, Dussault RG: Clinical evaluation of cervical facet joint infiltration. J Can Assoc Radiol 39: 118-120, 1988.

25. Bogduk N, Marsland A: The cervical zygapophysial joints as a source of neck pain. Spine 13: 610-617, 1988.

26. Hove B, Gyldensted C: Cervical analgesic facet joint arthrography. Neuroradiology 32: 456-459, 1990.

27. Bovim G, Berg R, Dale LG: Cervicogenic headache: anaesthetic blockade of cervical nerves (C2-C5) and facet joint (C2/C3). Pain 49: 315-320, 1992.

28. Aprill C, Bogduk N: The prevalence of cervical zygapophyseal joint pain: a first approximation. Spine 17: 744-747, 1992.

29. Busch E, Wilson PR: Atlanto-occipital and atlanto-axial injections in the treatment of headache and neck pain. Regional Anesth 14 (Suppl 2): 45, 1989.

30. Bogduk N: Local anaesthetic blocks of the second cervical ganglion: a technique with application in occipital headache. Cephalalgia 1: 41-50, 1981.

31. Lamer TJ: Ear pain due to cervical spine arthritis: treatment with cervical facet injection. Headache 31: 682-683, 1991.

32. Ehni GE, Benner B: Occipital neuralgia and the C1-2 arthrosis syndrome. J Neurosurg 61: 961-965, 1984.

33. Star MJ, Curd JG, Thorne RP: Atlantoaxial lateral mass osteoarthritis–a frequently overlooked cause of severe occipitocervical pain. Spine 17 (Suppl): S71-S76, 1992.

34. Barnsley L, Lord SM, Bogduk N: Comparative local anaesthetic blocks in the diagnosis of cervical zygapophysial joint pain. Pain 55: 99-106, 1993.

35. Barnsley L, Lord SM, Wallis BJ, Bogduk N: Chronic cervical zygapophysial joint pain after whiplash: a prospective prevalence study. Spine 20: 20-26, 1995.

36. Lord SM, Barnsley L, Wallis BJ, Bogduk N: Third occipital headache: a prevalence study. J Neurol Neurosurg Psychiatry 57: 1187-1190, 1994.

37. McCormick C: Arthrography of the atlanto-axial (C1-C2) joints: techniques and results. Journal of Interventional Radiology 2: 9-13, 1987.

38. Dreyfuss P, Roger J, Dreyer S, Fletcher D: Atlanto-occipital joint pain–a report of three cases and description of an intraarticular joint block technique. Regional Anesth 19: 344-351, 1994.

39. Kellgren JH: A preliminary account of referred pains arising from muscle. Br Med J 1: 325-327, 1938.

40. Bogduk N, Windsor M, Inglis A: The innervation of the cervical intervertebral discs. Spine 13: 2-8, 1988.

41. Bogduk N: The neurology of neck pain. International Journal of Pain Therapy 4: 68-78, 1994.

42. Friedenberg ZB, Miller WT: Degenerative disc disease of the cervical spine a comparative study of symptomatic and asymptomatic patients. J Bone Joint Surg Am 45-A: 1171-1178, 1963.

43. Heller CA, Stanley P, Lewis-Jones B, Heller RF: Value of X-Ray examinations of the cervical spine. Br Med J 287: 1276-1278, 1983.

44. Zapletal J, Hekster REM, Straver JS, Wilmink JT: Atlanto-odontoid osteoarthritis. Spine 20: 49-53, 1995.

45. Taylor JR: The pathology of neck sprain and cervical pain syndromes. International Journal of Pain Therapy 4: 91-99, 1994.

46. Barnsley L, Lord SM, Thomas P, Allen L, Southee A, Bogduk N: SPECT bone scans for the diagnosis of symptomatic cervical zygapophysial joints. Br J Rheumatol 32 Supp 2: 52, 1993. (Abstract)

47. Bogduk N: Headaches and cervical manipulation: a role in diagnosis. Patient Management 163-177, 1987.

48. Jull G, Bogduk N, Marsland A: The accuracy of manual diagnosis for cervical zygapophysial joint pain syndromes. Med J Aust 148: 233-236, 1988.

49. Okada K: Studies on the cervical facet joints using arthrography of the cervical facet joint. J Jap Orthop Ass 55: 563-580, 1981.

50. Dirheimer Y, Ramsheyi A, Reolon M: Positive arthrography of the craniocervical joints. Neuroradiology 12: 257-260, 1977.

51. Barnsley L, Bogduk N: Medial branch blocks are specific for the diagnosis of cervical zygapophysial joint pain. Regional Anesth 18: 343-350, 1993.

52. Voudouris NJ, Peck CL, Coleman G: Conditioned response models of placebo phenomena: further support. Pain 38: 109-116, 1989.

53. Peck C, Coleman G: Implications of placebo therapy for clinical research and practice in pain management. Theoretical Med 12: 247-270, 1991.

54. Bonica JJ, Butler SH: Local anaesthesia and regional blocks, Textbook of Pain. 3rd Ed. Edited by PD Wall, R Melzack. Churchill Livingston, Edinburgh, 1994, pp. 997-1023.

55. Bonica JJ, Buckley FP: Regional analgesia with local anesthetics, The Management of Pain. 2nd Ed. Edited by JJ Bonica. Lea & Febinger, Philadelphia, 1990, pp. 1883.

56. Boas RA: Nerve blocks in the diagnosis of low back pain. Neurosurg Clin 2: 807-816, 1991.

The Neck Disability Index:
Patient Assessment
and Outcome Monitoring in Whiplash

Howard Vernon

SUMMARY. Whiplash associated disorders have pain and disability affecting multiple systems. A key issue is to determine, however possible, those problems that lead to disability, since physical dysfunction has a major effect upon adjustments to life. The current study has taken the Oswestry Low Back Disability Index, and with adaptations that consider the neck and whiplash, and using current language and social issues, have developed a Neck Disability Index [NDI]. This self-report index has been tested reliable and valid as a measure of neck disability. The NDI has been shown to be a simple tool that could improve clinical assessments of whiplash; it is duplicated here, and its duplication and use is encouraged. *[Article copies available from The Haworth Document Delivery Service: 1-800-342-9678. E-mail address: getinfo@haworth.com]*

KEYWORDS. Whiplash, disability, questionnaire, index

Howard Vernon, DC, FCCS[C], is Associate Dean of Research, Canadian Memorial Chiropractic College, Toronto, Canada.

Address correspondence to: Howard Vernon, Canadian Memorial Chiropractic College, 1900 Bayview Avenue, Toronto, ON, M4G 3E6.

[Haworth co-indexing entry note]: "The Neck Disability Index: Patient Assessment and Outcome Monitoring in Whiplash." Vernon, Howard. Co-published simultaneously in *Journal of Musculoskeletal Pain* [The Haworth Medical Press, an imprint of The Haworth Press, Inc.] Vol. 4, No. 4, 1996, pp. 95-104; and: *Musculoskeletal Pain Emanating from the Head and Neck: Current Concepts in Diagnosis, Management and Cost Containment* [ed: Murray E. Allen] The Haworth Medical Press, an imprint of The Haworth Press, Inc., 1996, pp. 95-104. Single or multiple copies of this article are available from The Haworth Document Delivery Service [1-800-342-9678, 9:00 a.m. - 5:00 p.m. [EST]. E-mail address: getinfo@haworth.com].

INTRODUCTION

Injuries to the neck, and, in particular, those originating from a motor vehicle accident, constitute a significant burden to the health care system. Lifetime prevalence estimates for neck pain in general range from 45-71% (1,2,3), while the point prevalence has been reported at 9-12% (4).

Estimates of the incidence of whiplash-related injuries as reported in Barnsley et al. (5) range from 0.44 per 1000 (6) to 1.06 per 1000 (7). The recent Quebec Task Force Group [QTFG] (8) reported a one year incidence rate of whiplash claims in Quebec of 0.7 per 1000. Large differences between Canadian provinces were noted and thought to be due to differing tort law and compensation systems.

The degree to which whiplash-related symptoms persist in time appears variable in the reported literature. Norris and Watt (9) reported that 66% and 43% of their subjects continued to experience neck pain and headache respectively beyond six months post-accident. These figures are smaller in the report of Hildingsson and Toolanen (10), being 29% and 25%, respectively. The QTFG re-analyzed the data from Norris and Watt's study and found a trend toward persistence of neck pain and headache as the severity of initial presentation increased [i.e., from category 1 through 3]. Barnsley, Lord and Bogduk summarize the literature on chronicity by concluding that "between 14 and 42% of patients with whiplash injuries develop chronic neck pain and that approximately 10% will have constant severe pain indefinitely" (5).

Methods of determining both the clinical course of whiplash-related complaints and their impact upon the individual and society are rather crude. Most studies report symptom lists (8) but few have developed systematic symptom check lists. Outcomes such as claims data on length of disability, return to work and costs of claims are often used, and, although these data are useful to health policy analysts and insurers, they have less relevance to practicing clinicians. It was to address this need, i.e., for an instrument to assess what the QTFG was later to call "Whiplash-associated disorder (WAD)" that Vernon and Mior first developed the Neck Disability Index [NDI] (11).

THE NECK DISABILITY INDEX

The Neck Disability Index was modified [with permission] from the Oswestry Low Back Pain Disability Index [OLBPDI] of Fairbank et al. (12). The NDI, thus, has 10 items selected from the literature to have relevance to whiplash-associated disorder. Four items relate to subjective symptomatology, namely: "pain intensity," "headache," "concentration" and "sleeping." Four items relate to obligatory activities of daily living, namely: "lifting," "work," "driving," and "recreation." Two items, "personal care" and "reading" are discretionary activities of daily living. Items are scored on an ordinal scale from 0-5, with a maximum score of 50. The seminal study reported on 52 subjects, 70% of whom had suffered a whiplash-type injury within the past 4-6 weeks. Tables 1 and 2 display the mean item scores, ranks and alpha coefficients, and the range of total index scores, respectively.

The Index has good internal consistency [alpha = 0.80], while the total scores display a normal distribution, peaking in the moderately severe interval [15-24 out of 50]. In 17 subjects, test-retest reliability was determined using a two-day/no treatment interval as $R = 0.90$.

The NDI scores were found to correlate reasonably strongly with McGill Pain Questionnaire (13) scores [$R = 0.72$]. Finally, in order to determine the NDI's responsivity to change, change scores were compared to a visual analogue scale for improvement. The correlation coefficient was 0.60. The degree to which any of the subjects with a whiplash-type injury were receiving any disability benefits was not determined.

TABLE 1. Total Score and Item Reliability Analysis.

Item	Mean Score	Rank	Alpha
1. Pain intensity	1.70	6	0.79
2. Personal care	0.75	10	0.78
3. Lifting	2.20	2	0.78
4. Reading	2.10	4	0.78
5. Headache	2.60	1	0.84
6. Concentration	1.10	9	0.77
7. Work	1.50	7	0.76
8. Driving	2.00	5	0.76
9. Sleep	1.40	8	0.81
10. Recreation	2.20	3	0.77
Total Index = 0.80			

TABLE 2. Neck Disability: Frequency Plot of Total Scores.

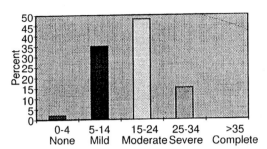

0-4	5-14	15-24	25-34	>35
None	Mild	Moderate	Severe	Complete

SUBSEQUENT STUDIES

In 1994, Hains et al. (14) reported on response set bias and internal factor structure of the NDI in 219 subjects with neck pain. After multivariate analysis of variance was conducted, no order or sequencing effect was detected. The internal consistency was determined by Cronbach's alpha at 0.90. The inter-item correlations ranged from $R = 0.31$ to 0.77, suggesting non-redundancy of items.

On factor analysis, one factor was extracted accounting for 59% of the variance, demonstrating that the NDI is, by and large, unidimensional. This factor was labelled "physical functioning." Factor weights were calculated and revealed no significant differences amongst the items. As such, it would seem that no inter-item weighting is required. Finally, a strong correlation between pain score [on a visual analog scale [VAS]] and NDI scores was found [$R = 0.70$].

Knaap et al. (15) reported on 46 subjects with neck pain. Test-retest reliability was high [ICC = 0.91, $P < 0.001$] as was internal consistency [Cronbach's alpha = 0.81]. As with the original report, no effect of age or gender was found.

Wallace et al. (16) used the NDI as an outcome measure in an uncontrolled study of 38 subjects with neck pain treated with spinal manipulation. The NDI scores were reduced from a mean of 19.3 ± 11.1 to 7.95 ± 5.76 [$P < 0.0001$]. The overall percentage change in NDI scores [over a 12 week period] was 58.8% which was nearly identical to the reduction in VAS pain scores [56%].

In recent unpublished work in our clinic (Vernon et al. unpublished) a high correlation has been observed between NDI scores in whiplash patients and scores on a new instrument–the Disability Rating Index (17). This finding further strengthens the concurrent validity of the NDI.

Vernon et al. (18) have recently reported on the NDI and the Oswestry Index in a sample of patients undergoing physical rehabilitation for work-related or motor-vehicle accident-related neck or back pain. A strong correlation R = 0.67, P = 0.018 was observed between change in disability index scores [NDI = 20] and a measure of patient satisfaction with the outcome of care [the Outcomes Satisfaction Index] (19).

CONCLUSION

Psychometric studies of the NDI have confirmed that it possesses high test-retest reliability, high internal consistency, a single-factor structure with only moderately high inter-item correlations making each item clinically and statistically useful. Clinical studies have confirmed good concurrent validity and good responsiveness. The NDI is a useful instrument for clinicians and researchers alike to employ in studies of whiplash-injured patients.

REFERENCES

1. Horal J: The clinical appearance of low back disorders in the city of Gothenburg, Sweden. Acta Orthop Scand Suppl 118:42-45, 1969.

2. Hult L: Cervical, dorsal and lumbar spinal syndromes. Acta Orthop Scand Suppl 17:175-277, 1954.

3. Hult L: The Munkfors Investigation: A study of the frequency and causes of stiff neck-brachialgia and lumbago-sciatic syndromes, as well as observations on certain signs and symptoms from the dorsal spine and the joints of the extremities in industrial and forest workers. Acta Orthop Scand Suppl 16:12-29, 1954.

4. Lawrence JS: Disc degeneration: its frequency and relationship to symptoms. Ann Rheum Dis 28: 121-137, 1969.

5. Barnsley L, Lord S, Bogduk N: Whiplash injury. Pain 58: 284-307, 1994.

6. Dvorak J, Valach L, Schmid, St: Cervical spine injuries in Switzerland. J Man Med 4:7-16, 1989.

7. Mills H and Horne G: Whiplash-manmade disease. NZ Med J 99:373-374, 1986.

8. Spitzer WO, Skovron ML, Salmi LR: Whiplash-Associated Disorders. Monograph of the Quebec Task Force on Whiplash Associated Disorders: Redefining "whiplash" and its management. Spine [Suppl 8S] 20, 1995.

9. Norris SH and Watt I: The prevalence of neck injuries resulting from rear-end collisions. J Bone Joint Surg, Br. 65: 608-611, 1983.

10. Hildingsson C and Toolanen G: Outcome after soft-tissue injury of the cervical spine: a prospective study of 93 car-accident victims. Acta Orthop Scand 61: 3576-359, 1990.

11. Vernon HT and Mior SA: The Neck Disability Index: a study of reliability and validity. J Manip Physiol Therap 14: 409-415, 1991.

12. Fairbank JCT, Couper J, Davies JB, O'Brien JP: The Oswestry low back pain disability index. Physiotherapy 66: 271-73, 1980.

13. Melzack R: The McGill Pain Questionnaire: major properties and scoring method. Pain 275-299, 1975.

14. Hains F, Waalen JK, Mior SA: Psychometric properties of the Neck Disability Index. In: Proc. 12th International Conference on Spinal Manipulation, Foundation for Chiropractic Education and Research, Palm Springs, 1994. pp. 8-9.

15. Knaap S, Langworthy J, Breen AC: The use of the Neck Disability Index in the evaluation of acute and chronic neck pain. in: Proc. 12th International Conference on Spinal Manipulation, Foundation for Chiropractic Education and Research, Palm Springs, 1994, p.10.

16. Wallace HL, Jahner S, Buckle K, Desai N: The relationship of changes in cervical curvature to VAS, NDI and pressure algometry in patients with neck pain. J Chiro Res Clin Inv 9: 19-23, 1994.

17. Salen B, Spangfort EV, Nygren A, Nordemar R: The Disability Rating Index: An instrument for the assessment of disability in clinical settings. J Clin Epidemiol 47: 1423-1434, 1994.

18. Vernon HT, Piccininni J, Kopansky-Giles D, Hagino C, Fuligni S: Chiropractic rehabilitation of spinal pain: principles, practices and outcomes data. J Can Chiro Assoc 39: 147-153, 1995.

19. Vernon HT, Miller R, Piccininni J, Fuligni S, Hagino C: Program evaluation in back care: development of an Outcomes Satisfaction Index. in: Proc. 4th World Federation of Chiropractic Congress, Washington DC, 1995.

NECK DISABILITY INDEX [NDI]

(Reformated with permission of authors © Vernon/Hagino 1987, for publication and distribution)

This questionnaire has been designed to give the doctor information as to how your neck pain has affected your ability to manage in everyday life. Please answer every section and mark in each section only the ONE box which applies to you. We realize you may consider that two of the statements in any one section relate to you, but please just mark the **one** box which most closely describes your problem.

Section 1–Pain Intensity
- ☐ I have no pain at the moment.
- ☐ The pain is very mild at the moment.
- ☐ The pain is moderate at the moment.
- ☐ The pain is fairly severe at the moment.
- ☐ The pain is very severe at the moment.
- ☐ The pain is the worst imaginable at the moment.

Section 2–Personal Care [Washing, Dressing, etc.]
- ☐ I can look after myself normally without causing extra pain.
- ☐ I can look after myself normally but it causes extra pain.
- ☐ It is painful to look after myself and I am slow and careful.
- ☐ I need some help but manage most of my personal care.
- ☐ I need help every day in most aspects of self care.
- ☐ I do not get dressed, I wash with difficulty and stay in bed.

NECK DISABILITY INDEX [NDI] [continued]

Section 3–Lifting
- ☐ I can lift heavy weights without extra pain.
- ☐ I can lift heavy weights but it gives me extra pain.
- ☐ Pain prevents me from lifting heavy weights off the floor, but I can manage if they are conveniently positioned, for example on a table.
- ☐ Pain prevents me from lifting heavy weights, but I can manage light to medium weights if they are conveniently positioned.
- ☐ I can lift very light weights.
- ☐ I cannot lift or carry anything at all.

Section 4–Reading
- ☐ I can read as much as I want to with no pain in my neck.
- ☐ I can read as much as I want to with slight pain in my neck.
- ☐ I can read as much as I want with moderate pain in my neck.
- ☐ I can't read as much as I want because of moderate pain in my neck.
- ☐ I can hardly read at all because of severe pain in my neck.
- ☐ I cannot read at all.

Section 5–Headaches
- ☐ I have no headaches at all.
- ☐ I have slight headaches which come infrequently.
- ☐ I have moderate headaches which come infrequently.
- ☐ I have moderate headaches which come frequently.
- ☐ I have severe headaches which come frequently.
- ☐ I have headaches almost all the time.

Section 6–Concentration

- ❏ I can concentrate fully when I want to with no difficulty.
- ❏ I can concentrate fully when I want to with slight difficulty.
- ❏ I have a fair degree of difficulty in concentrating when I want to.
- ❏ I have a lot of diffulty in concentrating when I want to.
- ❏ I have a great deal of difficulty in concentrating when I want to.
- ❏ I cannot concentrate at all.

Section 7–Work

- ❏ I can do as much work as I want to.
- ❏ I can only do my usual work, but no more.
- ❏ I can do most of my usual work, but no more.
- ❏ I cannot do my usual work.
- ❏ I can hardly do any work at all.
- ❏ I can't do any work at all.

Section 8–Driving

- ❏ I can drive my car without any neck pain.
- ❏ I can drive my car as long as I want with slight pain in my neck.
- ❏ I can drive my car as long as I want with moderate pain in my neck.
- ❏ I can't drive my car as long as I want because of moderate pain in my neck.
- ❏ I can hardly drive at all because of severe pain in my neck.
- ❏ I can't drive my car at all.

NECK DISABILITY INDEX [NDI] [continued]

Section 9–Sleeping
- ☐ I have no trouble sleeping.
- ☐ My sleep is slightly disturbed [less than 1 hr. sleepless].
- ☐ My sleep is mildly disturbed [1-2 hrs. sleepless].
- ☐ My sleep is moderately disturbed [2-3 hrs. sleepless].
- ☐ My sleep is greatly disturbed [3-5 hrs. sleepless].
- ☐ My sleep is completely disturbed [5-7 hrs. sleepless].

Section 10–Recreation
- ☐ I am able to engage in all my recreation activities with no neck pain at all.
- ☐ I am able to engage in all my recreation activities, with some pain in my neck.
- ☐ I am able to engage in most, but not all of my usual recreation activities because of pain in my neck.
- ☐ I am able to engage in a few of my usual recreation activities becuase of pain in my neck.
- ☐ I can hardly do any recreation activites because of pain in my neck.
- ☐ I can't do any recreation activities at all.

Dizziness, Imbalance, and Whiplash

Arthur I. Mallinson
Neil S. Longridge
Cindy Peacock

SUMMARY. Eighteen patients were evaluated for dizziness and imbalance resulting from whiplash associated disorder. Assessment consisted of standard caloric testing and Computerized Dynamic Posturography [CDP]. Although the standard vestibular tests showed no abnormalities in any of these patients, thirteen of them had abnormalities on CDP. The concept of dizziness is variously attributed to problems from the neck, brainstem or bloodflow to the brain and is ill defined in the literature. In our patients, efforts were made to delineate specifically the patient's complaints by careful history, which included anecdotal problems the patient reported that were recognized as possibly coming from the balance system of the inner ear. Dizziness may be attributable to a vestibular site of lesion, with the CDP results supporting a provisional diagnosis that somehow implicates the balance system of the inner ear. *[Article copies available from The Haworth Document Delivery Service: 1-800-342-9678. E-mail address: getinfo@haworth.com]*

Arthur I. Mallinson, MSc, is Neurophysiologist, Neil S. Longridge, MD, FRCS[C], is Medical Director, and Cindy Peacock, BSc, is Research Assistant, Neuro-otology Unit, Vancouver Hospital and Health Sciences Centre, University of British Columbia, Vancouver, Canada.

Address correspondence to: Dr. Neil Longridge, Division of Otolaryngology, 4th Floor, Willow Pavilion, Vancouver Hospital and Health Sciences Centre, 805 West 12th Avenue, Vancouver, BC, V5Z 1M9.

[Haworth co-indexing entry note]: "Dizziness, Imbalance, and Whiplash." Mallinson, Athur I., Neil S. Longridge, and Cindy Peacock. Co-published simultaneously in *Journal of Musculoskeletal Pain* [The Haworth Medical Press, an imprint of The Haworth Press, Inc.] Vol. 4, No. 4, 1996, pp. 105-112; and: *Musculoskeletal Pain Emanating from the Head and Neck: Current Concepts in Diagnosis, Management and Cost Containment* [ed: Murray E. Allen] The Haworth Medical Press, an imprint of The Haworth Press, Inc., 1996, pp. 105-112. Single or multiple copies of this article are available from The Haworth Document Delivery Service [1-800-342-9678, 9:00 a.m. - 5:00 p.m. [EST]. E-mail address: getinfo@haworth.com].

KEYWORDS. Whiplash, dizziness, imbalance, posturography

INTRODUCTION

In a rear end collision, the body accelerates forward while the head's inertia causes it to lag behind. The resulting extension ends when the soft tissues reach their limit of tension or compression, or when the head is stopped by the headrest of the vehicle. The head then rebounds forward, resulting in a flexion process. This is the motion of so-called whiplash, and is probably associated with extension, flexion, shear, tension, compression, and possibly other features yet to be elucidated (1).

McNab (2) showed that there was significant injury to the peri-vertebral musculature in serious whiplash injuries. Prognostic indicators appeared to be the severity of early symptoms including radicular symptomatology of the neck.

Dizziness is often mentioned as a symptom in whiplash associated disorder [WAD] (1,3,4,5). The etiology of vertigo, dizziness and imbalance may be due to stretching of the ligaments in the cervical spine, irritation or damage to the vertebral arterial blood supply and damage to the autonomic nervous system in the cervical spine (5,6). Damage to the inner ear is also a possibility (1,7).

The incidence of dizziness in WAD has been quoted as 21% (4) to 85% (1). The aim of the present paper was to elicit from patients the specific dizzy-related complaints of which they suffer. Patients' complaints were compared to results of standardly recognized balance assessment techniques of electronystagmography [ENG] and Computerized Dynamic Posturography [CDP].

It has been observed that some patients have subjective vague complaints of lightheadedness, unsteadiness, and dislike of things moving rapidly past them, particularly in malls, supermarkets or at the edge of a busy road. Fluorescent lighting may be distressing and checkered floors may be bothersome. Visual vestibular mismatch is a recognized syndrome where it is assumed that vestibular input and ocular input do not mesh precisely, resulting in symptomatic awareness of particular difficulties. Excessive nausea and motion sickness are frequent complaints. Although dizziness often resolves, prolonged symptomatology sometimes persists. The current treatment for dizziness is vestibular rehabilitation exercises of the Cawthorne-Cooksey (8,9) variety, but the rehabilitation process for dizziness is sometimes limited by concomitant neck pain. In more severe WAD, some patients may be incapacitated for a prolonged period and may not complain of vertiginous symptoms until several weeks after the accident, at a time when they move around enough to become aware of their difficulty. This might account for some of the short delays in apparent dizziness onset following whiplash trauma.

Patients and Methods

This retrospective review was obtained by reviewing motor vehicle accident charts of patients seen by one investigator [NSL], including ENG and CDP data from the preceding three years. Only rear end accidents were included. Pedestrians and patients involved with side swipe or head on collisions were excluded. Patients who had a head injury were excluded. There was no random selection and no control group. Patient assessment consisted of history, otolaryngological and balance physical examination, ENG, audiometry and CDP assessment using EquiTest™ protocol. The ENG (10) protocol included assessment for spontaneous nystagmus with eyes open and eyes closed, gaze nystagmus, optokinetic nystagmus and smooth pursuit. Caloric-induced nystagmus was also assessed, including fixation suppression ratio. Postural testing as described by Barber (11) was not undertaken as it had not been found to be helpful in a study of non-traumatic vertiginous patients (12). The CDP protocol followed exactly the EquiTest™ interpretation manual (13). The Sensory Organization Test [SOT] sequence used in this protocol has been described elsewhere (14).

RESULTS

The charts of 77 patients who had sustained motor vehicle accident injuries were examined. Only 18 patients [Table 1] were pure rear end accidents. All but one were wearing a seat belt. All but one of them had sought medical attention from either their family doctor or a hospital Emergency Ward.

Computerized Dynamic Posturography was abnormal in 13 of 18 patients. In 11 of these 13 patients the abnormality was a specific pattern of abnormality which suggests impairment in the vestibular system. In particular there was poor performance on SOT conditions 5 and/or 6. Two patients had a more generalized abnormality pattern which we have come to assume indicates mild inability to integrate sensory information of balance.

Eight patients had characteristic vestibular syndromes [Table 1] (15): benign positional vertigo, acute vestibulopathy [vestibular neuronitis], recurrent vestibulopathy. Seven of these eight had abnormal posturography patterns, with five of the seven being specific vestibular abnormality patterns.

TABLE 1. Subject Profiles and Responses to Testing.

PATIENT	SUBJECTIVE COMPLAINTS	ONSET LATENCY	EQUITEST
1. [38F]	spinning, lightheaded imbalance, blurred vision	immediately after #2 signif incr with #3	abnormal vestibular
2. [54M]	feel drunk constantly worse with head movement	<30 days	grossly abnormal nonspecific
3. [33M]	nausea with head movement lightheaded	30 minutes	abnormal vestibular
4. [18F]	nausea vague imbalance	6 days	normal
5. [42F]	unsteady, clumsy, might fall like being on a merry-go-round	not known	abnormal vestibular
6. [60M]	like a drunk, blurry vision, feel funny in malls	3 days	abnormal vestibular
7. [28F]	spinning for a week, trouble bike riding down hills	minutes	abnormal vestibular
8. [46M]	feel seasick, unsteady if I get up fast	3 days	normal
9. [29F]	"sea legs," nausea, woozy imbalance, pull to left	7-14 days	abnormal vestibular
10. [28F]	must focus when I walk motion sickness	<1 day	abnormal vestibular
11. [45F]	walks like a drunk, nausea trouble in malls, not secure	90 days	abnormal vestibular
12. [48M]	like being on a merry-go-round nausea waves, wobbly	2-3 days	abnormal vestibular
13. [39F]	2 one hour spells of spinning brief spins with movement	<1 day	abnormal vestibular
14. [30F]	"sea legs" also lightheaded	30 days	abnormal nonspecific
15. [53F]	imbalance, like looking at water trouble in malls and on stairs	immediate	normal
16. [49M]	whirling, eyes jiggle imbalance, nausea	1 day	abnormal vestibular
17. [40M]	lightheaded, nausea spin when I look up	4 days	normal
18. [33F]	veering, unsteady "like stepping off an elevator"	<1 day	normal

DISCUSSION

The concept of vestibular involvement in whiplash injury is poorly discussed in the literature pertaining to cervical spine injury. Although true vertigo is alluded to, we only heard the complaint in eight of our patients, allowing us to make a definitive diagnosis in all eight. We felt that ten patients who denied true vertigo had problems with the vestibular system as supported by the posturography results. A combination of posturography and a very careful history taking is crucial to delineate the problem as coming from the vestibular system.

Hinokee (5) found 87% of patients involved in a flexion extension injury had dizziness whereas it was a much smaller percentage in a study by Sturzenegger (4). Table 1 lists complaints voiced by patients in describing their symptoms. Previous papers, presumably for reasons of simplicity have grouped patients with these complaints as being dizzy, lightheaded or imbalanced. A main purpose of this paper is to draw attention to the fact that, if questioned, many patients with vestibular disease other than WAD also voice complaints mentioned in Table 1. The complaints therefore arise from an abnormality in the balance system.

Although poorly understood, it may be that the differing functions of the vestibular system are managed by discrete parts of the system. This is suggested by the fact that certain "unusual complaints" are described characteristically in a markedly similar fashion by some patients and denied by others. For instance, persistent imbalance [8/18 patients], inability to tolerate excessive optokinetic stimulation [7/18 patients], "feeling drunk" [6/18 patients], and "sealegs" [4/18 patients] are common complaints. However, attempts to delineate a common thread in these groups, or use the complaints as predictors of examination or test results have been unsuccessful.

Ten patients did not have classical vestibular syndromes but had complaints which suggested an abnormality in the balance system. Interestingly six of these patients had abnormal posturography suggestive of a vestibular abnormality pattern.

Sixteen of 18 patients showed no abnormality on ENG. There was no evidence of spontaneous nystagmus greater than 7° per second, no gaze nystagmus, smooth pursuit abnormality, or optokinetic abnormality noted. There was no caloric abnormality detected in any of the patients. In two patients there was evidence of nystagmus characteristic for benign positional vertigo on position testing. These findings are in significant contradistinction to those of Oosterveld (1) who found significant ENG abnormalities in many patients who were tested after a whiplash.

Computerized Dynamic Posturography may detect abnormalities in patients with vestibular disease when ENG is normal (14). The most useful test was CDP which was abnormal in 13 of 18 patients, all but two of the 13 abnormalities showing a pattern characteristic for inner ear vestibular disease. As Chester (7) found from the legal investigative standpoint, CDP is more frequently abnormal than ENG. Computerized Dynamic Posturography shows a characteristic configuration for normal and abnormal. Normal CDP results occurred in our series despite symptoms of WAD.

Most dizzy patients show neutral or improved function by Cawthorne-Cooksey rehabilitation exercises. In some patients who have flexion extension injury, not only are they not improved they may be distinctly worse. In our study two patients were symptomatically worse following these exercises. Some patients will demonstrate this in physical terms by stating that their symptoms are very severe the next day, following a day of activity.

Under normal circumstances, there are two main reflexes mediated by the vestibular system utilizing all the afferent information. The vestibulo-ocular reflex [VOR] serves to foveate an image on the back of the eye. Operation of this reflex can be indicated using a simple doll's eye maneuver. The efficiency of the reflex can be utilized using bedside testing (16) or by caloric tests. The vestibulospinal reflexes [VSR] or "righting" reflexes serve to orient a patient in space with respect to the surroundings and to earth vertical. Patients can often be separated by history as having an abnormality affecting one or the other reflex. For instance a patient complaining solely of imbalance could be thought of having a VSR impairment, while a patient complaining of intolerance to a patterned rug or to excessive movement in the visual field could be delineated as having a VOR complaint. By this delineation, 9 of our series [50%] had a VSR type of abnormality, 4 had a VOR problem, and 5 had features suggestive of both groups. No other differences could be found among the three groups.

While two patients had generalized abnormalities of balance on posturography, the observation of a specific abnormality pattern in SOT five and/or six in 11 of our patients with WAD allows us to speculate strongly that the inner ear may be the cause of the vestibular compromise in many of these patients, although the presence of visual vestibular mismatch could indicate the possibility of a more central component or a combination of inner ear and central disease.

If we assume that acute trauma has its clinical effects soon after application, then if the vestibular system was damaged in a whiplash event, then some dizzy type symptoms should have their presentation soon after the traumatic event. Among the 18 subjects in this study, 13 had onset within one week, five were delayed in onset by over seven days. Among the early onset subjects, eight had positive CDP and five negative. Among the delayed onset subjects, all five had positive CDP test results that might suggest some vestibular mechanisms for their symptoms. The delay in onset of dizziness is assumed, without proof, to be due to the fact that a patient who is markedly incapacitated becomes aware of symptoms as pain eases and mobility returns.

CONCLUSIONS

Eighteen post-whiplash patients with complaints of dizziness were retrospectively analyzed using sophisticated CDP which found a high incidence of positive findings suggestive of a vestibular disturbance. In the same patients, there was a low incidence of findings of vestibular disturbance using standard ENG. There was no correlation between positive CDP findings and early symptom onset, with many of the early onset patients having negative CDP, and all of the delayed onset having positive CDP. In most of the patients with CDP abnormalities, the pattern of abnormality suggested that the inner ear was the likely cause of the disorder. In those with a nonspecific pattern of abnormality and those with normal CDP, the site was unknown and could be central, from the inner ear, or from the neck.

REFERENCES

1. Oosterveld WJ, Kortschot HW, Kingma GG, et al.: Electronystagmographic findings following cervical whiplash injuries. Acta Otolaryngologica Stockholm 111: 201-205, 1991.

2. MacNab I: Acceleration injuries of the cervical spine. J Bone Joint Surg 46-A: 1797-1799, 1964.

3. Lee J, Giles K, Drummond P: Psychological disturbances and an exaggerated response to pain in patients with whiplash injury. J Psychosomatic Res 37(2): 105-110, 1993.

4. Sturzenegger M, DiStefano G, Radanov BP, et al.: Presenting symptoms and signs after whiplash injury: the influence of accident mechanisms. Neurology 44: 688-693, 1994.

5. Hinoki M. Vertigo due to whiplash injury: a neurotological approach. Acta Otolaryngologica Stockholm 419(Suppl): 9-29, 1985.

6. Pfaltz CR: Vertigo in disorders of the neck. in Vertigo. Dix MR and Hood JD (Eds) 1984. John Wiley & Sons Ltd. Chichester.

7. Chester JB: Whiplash, postural control and the inner ear. Spine 16(7): 716-720, 1991.

8. Cawthorne TE: Vestibular injuries. Proc R Soc Med (Lond) 39: 270-273, 1945.

9. Cooksey FS: Rehabilitation in vestibular injuries. Proc R Soc Med (Lond) 38: 273-275, 1945.

10. Barber HO, Stockwell CW: Manual of electronystagmography. 2nd. ed.: C.V. Mosby Company. St. Louis, 1980.

11. Barber HO: Positional nystagmus especially after head injury. Laryngoscope 74: 891-944, 1964.

12. Longridge NS, Barber HO: Bilateral paroxysmal positioning nystagmus. J. Otol. 7(5), 395-400, 1978.

13. Neurocom International Inc. EquiTest Interpretation Manual 1992. Neurocom International, Clackamas, OR.

14. Lipp M, Longridge NS: Computerized Dynamic Posturography: its place in evaluation of the patient with dizziness and imbalance. J Otolaryngology 23(3): 177-183, 1994.

15. Longridge NS, Robinson RG: Approach to the patient with dizziness and vertigo. In Textbook of Internal Medicine, Kelley WN (ed). 2nd edition, 1992: JB Lippincott, Philadelphia.

16. Longridge NS, Mallinson AI: A discussion of the Dynamic Illegible "E" Test. A new method of screening for aminoglycoside ototoxicity. Otol Head Neck Surg 92(6): 671-677, 1984.

Manipulation and Mobilization of the Cervical Spine: The Results of a Literature Survey and Consensus Panel

Ian Coulter

SUMMARY. Objectives: To review the scientific evidence for both manipulation and mobilization therapies for the cervical spine. This report presents the results from a review of the medical, chiropractic, osteopathic, physical therapy, and dental literature on the efficacy, complications, and indications for manipulation and mobilization of the cervical spine, and the appropriateness ratings of indications for manipulation and mobilization.

Ian Coulter, PhD, is Health Consultant, RAND; Adjunct Professor, School of Dentistry, UCLA; Research Professor, Los Angeles College of Chiropractic; and Behavioral Scientist, Sepuleveda Veteran's Hospital Administration Medical Center, Los Angeles, CA.

Address correspondence to: Dr. Ian Coulter, RAND, 1700 Main Street, P.O. Box 2138, Santa Monica, CA 90406-2138.

The authors wish to acknowledge the contribution of Paul Shekelle, MD, PhD, Alan Adams, DC, Eric Hurwitz, MS, DC, William Meeker, DC, Dan Hansen, DC, Robert Mootz, DC, and Peter Aker, DC.

The research on which this article is based was funded by the Consortium for Chiropractic Research and was a joint project involving RAND, the Los Angeles College of Chiropractic, and the Palmer College of Chiropractic West.

The opinions expressed are those of the author.

[Haworth co-indexing entry note]: "Manipulation and Mobilization of the Cervical Spine: The Results of a Literature Survey and Consensus Panel." Coulter, Ian. Co-published simultaneously in *Journal of Musculoskeletal Pain* [The Haworth Medical Press, an imprint of The Haworth Press, Inc.] Vol. 4, No. 4, 1996, pp. 113-123; and: *Musculoskeletal Pain Emanating from the Head and Neck: Current Concepts in Diagnosis, Management and Cost Containment* [ed: Murray E. Allen] The Haworth Medical Press, an imprint of The Haworth Press, Inc., 1996, pp. 113-123. Single or multiple copies of this article are available from The Haworth Document Delivery Service [1-800-342-9678, 9:00 a.m. - 5:00 p.m. [EST]. E-mail address: getinfo@haworth.com].

Methods: Articles were identified through searches of computerized databases [MEDLINE [*Index Medicus*], CHIROLARS [*Chiropractic Literature Analyses and Retrieval System*] etc.], review of article's bibliographies, and advice from experts. This yielded 362 primary articles on cervical spine manual therapy and 145 articles on complications. Priority was given to research that used randomized, controlled trial [RCT] designs. Second priority was given to non-experimental studies including cohort, case-control, and cross sectional studies. Case series and case reports were given lowest priority. This process produced 108 studies [16 RCTs; 13 cohort; 27 case series; 52 case reports]. A panel of nine experts were provided with the literature review and were then used to complete two rounds of ratings for appropriateness of indications for manipulation and mobilization. The panel was multidisciplinary in composition.

Results: 1. Literature Review. The review provided 67 articles on efficacy; 14 RCTs. For acute neck pain there were three RCTs for mobilization but only one for manipulation. Results varied but mobilization is probably better than collar and rest, but exercises are equally effective and the one trial of manipulation showed an immediate improvement that was not sustained at one week. For subacute and chronic neck pain there was one RCT for mobilization and four for manipulation. Results show short-term pain relief and motion enhancement. A small but significantly significant outcome was shown for manipulation compared to physiotherapy. For headache there were five RCTs, 10 case series, 19 case reports of manipulation, and one RCT for mobilization. For muscle tension headaches the data support but do not prove that manipulation and/or mobilization may provide short-term relief for some patients. Evidence for long-term benefit is less conclusive. For migraine, one RCT and five other studies for manipulation were reviewed. The literature neither supports nor refutes manipulation/mobilization for migraine. For shoulder/arm/hand pain; thoracic outlet syndrome, carpel tunnel, temporomandibular joint [TMJ] disorders; blood pressure and heart rate, cervical spine/intersegmental motion, cervical spine curvature, miscellaneous conditions, there is insufficient evidence to refute or support either manipulation or mobilization. Articles document 110 cases of complications published in English relating to manipulation. The vast majority involved vertebrobasilar accidents [VBA]. Based on the available evidence we estimate the rate of complications to be 1 per million manipulations.

2. Panel Ratings. The panel rated 1,436 indications [clinical scenarios of patients who might be considered for cervical manipulation or mobilization] in the final round, with disagreement on 2% of the indications. They rated 43% as inappropriate for manipulation or mobilization. Appropriate and uncertain indications accounted for

16% and 41%, respectively. The frequency with which indications occur in a population is unknown and therefore the rate of inappropriate manipulation/mobilization being rendered to patients cannot be determined at this time. *[Article copies available from The Haworth Document Delivery Service: 1-800-342-9678. E-mail address: getinfo@haworth.com]*

KEYWORDS. Manipulation, mobilization, cervical spine

INTRODUCTION

Spinal manipulation and mobilization are used as a treatment modality for an array of conditions, including back pain, neck pain, headache, and other somatic and non-somatic conditions. Neck and headache pain are second only to back pain as the most common reason for providing manipulative therapy. Data from the utilization of chiropractic services (1) suggest that chiropractors alone provide between 18 to 38 million cervical manipulations per year for neck pain and headaches. Other providers [e.g., osteopaths, physical therapists, medical manual therapists] also provide such services. The purpose of this review is to assess the evidence for the use of cervical spine manipulation and mobilization for the treatment of a range of conditions, primarily neck pain and headache, and to document the complications resulting from its use. Spinal manipulation, for the purpose of this review, refers to the use of a controlled, judiciously applied dynamic thrust [adjustment, that may include combined extension and rotation of the upper cervical spinal segments], applied with high or low velocity and low amplitude force directed at the spinal joint segment within patient tolerance. These procedures often take joints into the "paraphysiological" space resulting in joint cavitation. Mobilization is defined as a controlled, judiciously applied force of low velocity and variable amplitude directed to spinal joint segment[s]. These procedures usually do not take joints beyond the passive range of motion and do not result in joint cavitation.

METHODS

The study employed a University of California at Los Angeles [RAND/ UCLA] consensus panel methodology to investigate the appropriateness of cervical manipulation and mobilization [this method has been extensively described elsewhere] (2,3) and an explicit literature based method employing a panel of nine clinical experts. The process used in this study is a modified delphi in which the panel of experts rates sets of indications on two separate occasions. The first set of ratings is conducted by the panelists individually following their reading of the literature review provided to them. The second set of ratings occur in a panel meeting where the experts review and discuss their first ratings.

The panel was a multidisciplinary one consisting of 4 chiropractors, 4 medical physicians, and 1 individual who is qualified in both chiropractic and medicine. The panel was chosen to ensure a geographic distribution and varied clinical expertise. It included 2 surgeons, 2 neurologists, 1 family physician, 2 chiropractic specialists, and 2 chiropractic general practitioners.

The consensus method begins with a systematic literature review. Structured database searching of four computerized bibliographic databases: MEDLINE [*Index Medicus*], EMBASE [*Exerpta Medica*], CHIRO-LARS [*Chiropractic Literature Analysis and Retrieval System*], CINAHL [*Cumulative Index of Nursing and Allied Health Literature*]. This was performed to identify English-only citations from 1966 to the present. Databases with later start dates were searched from the earliest possible time. Searching of these four databases allowed for the retrieval of citations from mainstream medicine in North America and Europe, allopathic medicine, chiropractic, osteopathic, physiotherapy, nursing, and dental temporomandibular joint [TMJ] literature. This search yielded 1,457 citations, of which 705 were identified as relevant.

After further review for relevance this search yielded 362 primary articles on cervical spine manual therapy and 145 articles on complications for a total of 507 articles. In addition two unpublished random controlled trials [RCTs] were included. Priority for review was given to RCTs, followed by non-experimental studies, including cohort, case-control, and cross sectional studies. Case series and case studies were given the lowest priority. This ranking generated 108 studies or reports that were judged to deal with efficacy: 16 RCTs, 13 cohort studies, 27 case series, and 52 case reports. These were reviewed and rated by two independent investigators using criteria taken from the work by Koes (4). There were several major limitations encountered in the literature review. Firstly, the studies are of variable quality. The range of rating scores for the studies was 33-77 out of a possible 100 with the majority receiving a score of less than 50. Secondly, they differ in the outcomes that were assessed. Thirdly, the study populations varied [differing symptoms, differing prognoses, etc.]. Fourthly, the type of manipulation and mobilization used varied among the studies. Fifthly, as a result of the above, it was impossible to combine the results of the studies.

The literature review and the set of indications derived from the literature and informed sources was circulated to the panelists to be rated individually for appropriateness [described below] for manipulation and mobilization. The panel of experts was then convened to rate the same indications for the cervical spine following reporting and discussion of the previous ratings.

RESULTS–LITERATURE REVIEW (5)

Neck Pain. Five RCTs, 1 cohort study, 4 case series, and 24 case reports were identified that attempted to assess the effectiveness of cervical spine manipulation for the treatment of neck pain. An additional 4 RCTs, 1 cohort study, and 1 case series dealt, at least in part, with the effectiveness of mobilization for neck pain. The manipulation RCTs focused primarily on subacute and chronic pain, while four of the mobilization RCTs addressed acute pain.

Acute Neck Pain. There was one RCT presenting data about the efficacy of cervical spine manipulation specifically for patients with acute neck pain. It reported a statistically significant improvement in pain relief for patients treated with manipulation or muscle relaxant compared to patients treated with a muscle relaxant alone. The limited literature available on mobilization for acute neck pain indicates that it may be beneficial for some patients, at least compared to rest and cervical collar, although instruction on mobilization and exercises may be equally beneficial.

Subacute and Chronic Neck Pain. Four RCTs of manipulation and one RCT of mobilization for subacute or chronic neck pain were reviewed. Seven other studies provided additional data. There is evidence from the literature that cervical spine manipulation and/or mobilization may provide at least short-term pain relief and range of motion enhancement for persons with subacute or chronic neck pain. The published results are insufficient to make efficacy determinations separately for patients with subacute pain and patients with chronic neck pain.

Headache. Five RCTs, 10 case series, and 19 case reports were identified that assessed the effectiveness of cervical spine manipulation for headache. One additional RCT addressed, in part, the effectiveness of mobilization techniques for headache.

Muscle Tension Headache. Four RCTs of manipulation and one RCT of mobilization for headache were reviewed. Nine other studies provided additional data. The literature is sparse but suggests that cervical spine manipulation and/or mobilization may provide short-term relief for some patients with muscle tension [and other non-migraine] headaches. The evidence for long-term benefit is much less conclusive.

Migraine Headache. One RCT of manipulation for migraine headache and five other studies were reviewed. The literature is too limited to support or refute the use of cervical spine manipulation and/or mobilization for patients suffering from migraine headaches.

Shoulder/Arm/Hand Pain: Acute, Subacute, and Chronic Pain. The literature is insufficient to support or refute the use of cervical spine manipulation and/or mobilization for patients with pain of the shoulder, arm, and/or hand of any duration based on data from a single RCT and two case series.

Thoracic Outlet Syndrome, Carpel Tunnel Syndrome, Temporomandibular Joint Disorders. There are no RCTs for any of these conditions for manipulation or mobilization. Isolated case reports record clinical improvement in some patients.

Blood Pressure and Heart Rate, Cervical Spine/Intersegmental Motion, Cervical Spine Curvature, Miscellaneous Conditions. There is insufficient evidence to support or refute the use of cervical spine mobilization or manipulation for most of the above entities. However, the literature does provide evidence that manipulation of the cervical spine increases range of motion and intersegmental mobility. The clinical significance of this is not known.

Complications. Articles documenting more than 110 cases of complications allegedly arising from cervical spine manipulation have been published in English. The vast majority of these complications involved vertebrobasilar accidents [VBA] with consequences such as brainstem and/or cerebellar infarction, Wallenberg's Syndrome [obstruction of the posterior inferior cerebellar artery], and Locked-In Syndrome [occlusion of basilar artery]. Other reported complications include spinal cord compression, vertebral fracture, tracheal rupture, diaphragm paralysis, internal carotid hematoma, and cardiac arrest.

It is difficult to estimate the frequency of vertebrobasilar accidents and other complications among patients undergoing cervical spine manipulation because of the uncertainty of both caseload and the number of cervical manipulations that patients receive over a specified period of time. There were no serious neurological complications during one year among 460 providers and approximately 150,000 cervical manipulations in one large case series. Based on the best available evidence we estimate the rate of complications as a result of cervical spine manipulation to be one per million manipulations.

Expert Panel Ratings for Appropriateness

The project staff compiled the initial indications list, using the literature review, the advice of chiropractors, medical physicians, and physical therapists. The indications categorized persons in terms of their history, symptoms, physical and radiographic findings, and response to prior treatment. Each indication can be considered to represent a clinical scenario of a patient that may present to a clinician's office. We attempted to compile lists that were detailed, comprehensive, and manageable. The lists needed enough detail so that patients presenting with a particular indication would be relatively homogeneous, in the sense that doing the procedure would be equally appropriate [or inappropriate] for all of them. We sought to include all indications for doing cervical manipulation or mobilization that might arise in practice. At the same time, we tried to keep the total number of indications low enough to allow the panelists to rate all of them within a reasonable length of time.

The indications were organized into 13 "chapters" which clustered indications within major symptoms or primary problems. For example the first two chapters were as follows:

1. Acute neck pain and signs of painful and/or limited active range of motion and anatomically consistent with a musculotendinous distribution and no radiculopathy.
2. Subacute or chronic neck pain and signs of painful and/or limited active range of motion and pain anatomically consistent with a musculotendinous distribution and no radiculopathy.

The instructions asked the panelists to use their own best clinical judgment considering an average group of patients presenting to an average physician who performed manipulation and mobilization and to rank the appropriateness of manipulation or mobilization on 1 to 9 scale. Appropriate care was defined to mean that expected health benefits to the patient [e.g., increased life expectancy, relief of symptoms, reduction of anxiety, improved functional capacity, etc.] exceeded expected health risks [e.g., mortality, morbidity, pain produced by the procedure] by a sufficiently wide margin that the procedure is worth doing. Extremely appropriate indications were rated 9, extremely inappropriate 1, and indications for which the risks and benefits were about equal [or unknown] were rated a 5. The instructions also included definitions of important terms. For each indication, the median was used to measure the central tendency of the nine panelists' ratings and the mean absolute distance from the median to measure the dispersion of the ratings. Table 1 shows the median ratings of the indications by the panel of experts for rounds one and two and the percent of agreement. Our preferred definition of agreement is that after discarding one extreme high and one extreme low rating, the remaining seven fall within any three-point range. According to this definition, at the conclusion of the process, panelists agreed on the ratings in 40% of the indications. Our preferred definition of disagreement is that, after discarding one extreme high and one extreme low rating, at least one of the remaining seven falls in the lowest three point region [1 to 3] and at least one falls in the highest. Table 1 shows that the panelists disagreed on the ratings in only 2% of the indications on the final round.

There was an increase in agreement [from 20% to 40%] and a decrease in disagreement [from 10% to 2%] between the initial round and the final round. The final round rated 1,436 indications. For comparison, in an earlier study on manipulation only of the lumbar spine, using the same definition for disagreement, a similar multidisciplinary panel of experts had disagreement on 3% of 1,550 indications.

It is also of some interest to examine the number of indications that were rated inappropriate. Each indication falls into one of three categories of appropriateness: inappropriate, uncertain, or appropriate. An indication was called "appropriate" if the panelists assigned a median rating in the 7 to 9 range without disagreement, and it was "inappropriate" if they assigned a 1 to 3 rating without disagreement. We classified an indication as "uncertain" for either of two reasons. The benefits and risk of doing the procedure were considered roughly the same [a median rating of 4 to 6], or the panelists disagreed on the proper rating. Table 2 categorizes the final indications by their appropriateness ratings.

Forty-three percent of indications were rated inappropriate. Appropriate and uncertain indications each accounted for 16% and 41% of the total, respectively. Table 2 represents aggregate values for both manipulation and mobilization. Table 3 compares the results for manipulation and mobilization. Comparing the results in Table 3 it is clear that more indications

TABLE 1. Median Rating, Percentage of Agreement to Expert Panel.

ITEM	Initial round	Final round
Number Of Indications	1171	1436
Average Median	4.60	4.02
Mean Absolute Deviation From The Median	1.51	1.14
% Of Agreement	19.98%	39.97%
% Of Disagreement	10.08%	2.09%

TABLE 2. Categories of Appropriateness of 1,436 Indications for Cervical Manipulation.

CATEGORY	Number of indications	Indications %
Inappropriate	623	43%
Uncertain	586	41%
Appropriate	122	16%

TABLE 3. Categories of Appropriateness of Indications for Cervical Manipulation and Mobilization.

Category	MANIPULATION		MOBILIZATION	
	# Of Indications	% Of Indications	# Of Indications	% Of Indications
Inappropriate	424	57.6%	199	28.4%
Uncertain	230	31.3%	356	50.9%
Appropriate	82	11.1%	145	20.7%
Total	736	100%	700	100%

were rated as inappropriate for manipulation than for mobilization and that the category of "uncertain" was largest for mobilization. The level of disagreement also differed for manipulation and mobilization. For mobilization the panel disagreed on 0.9% of the indications while for manipulation they disagreed on 3.3%.

The low average median and large number of indications rated inappropriate do not necessarily suggest inappropriate care is being rendered. It may be the case that in practice, manipulation or mobilization is used for highly appropriate indications. It will require the collection of clinically detailed patient level data on persons presenting with symptoms referable to the cervical spine to understand the frequency of appropriate use of clinical spine mobilization and manipulation.

Although it is not possible to report on the results of all the chapters rated by the panel, the clinical factors for neck pain being rated as appropriate for manipulation included: pain anatomically consistent with musculotendinous distribution; no evidence of radiculopathy; no contraindication for manipulation. Clinical factors for acute/subacute headache being rated as appropriate for manipulation included: normal neurological history/physical examination; no contraindications on cervical radiographs. For chronic headache they included: non-throbbing headache with no prodrome; no clinical risk factors; no radiographic contraindications. Clinical factors associated with indications rated as inappropriate for manipulation included: presence of clinical substantial trauma for neck pain in the absence of radiographs; presence of clinical risk factors in the absence of radiographs; presence of radiographic contraindications; presence of disc herniation or spinal canal stenosis. The clinical factors associated with appropriate and inappropriate indications for cervical spine mobilization were in general the same as those for manipulation although in almost all the indications the use of mobilization was rated more favorably than manipulation. The one clinical factor which was much different for mobilization vis-a-vis manipulation was the presence of possible or definite radiculopathy, which was a more negative factor for manipulation than for mobilization.

CONCLUSION

The results of the literature review support, but do not prove, that cervical manipulation or mobilization provide at least short-term benefit to some patients with neck pain and headache. A multidisciplinary group of clinical experts, starting with the literature synthesis and supplementing it with their clinical judgment, were able to agree that for certain patient presentations, cervical spine manipulation or mobilization was appropriate, that is, the expected benefit exceeded the expected risk. This panel also identified patient presentations that were inappropriate for these procedures, and in addition identified a large number of patient presentations for which, even using their best clinical judgment, the risks and benefits are uncertain. Until the results of new clinical trials are available these criteria provide a useful framework for clinicians to judge which patients might be offered cervical manipulation or mobilization as a therapeutic option.

REFERENCES

1. Shekelle PG, Brook RH: A community based study of the use of chiropractic services. Am J Public Health 81:439-442,1991.

2. Park RE, Fink A, Brook RH, Chassin MR, Merrick N, Kosekoff J, Solomon DH: Physician ratings of appropriate indications for six medical and surgical procedures. Am J Public Health 76: 766-772,1986.

3. Brook RH: The RAND/UCLA appropriateness method. In McCormach KA, Moore SR, Siegel RA (eds): Clinical Practice Guideline Development. Methodology Perspectives. US Department of Health and Human Services, AHCPR; 1994:59-65.

4. Koes BW, Bouter LM, Knipshild PG, Van Mameren H, et al.: The effectiveness of manual therapy, physiotherapy and continued treatment by the general practitioner for chronic nonspecific back and neck complaints: design of a randomized clinical trial. J Manipulative Physiol Ther 14(9): 498-502,1991.

5. Coulter ID, Shekelle PG, Mootz RD, Hansen DT: The use of expert panel results: The RAND panel for appropriateness of manipulation and mobilization of the cervical spine. Topics Clinical Chiropractic 2(3):54-62,1995.

The Pros and Cons
of Passive Physical Therapy Modalities
for Neck Disorders

Alain-Y. Bélanger

SUMMARY. Objectives: To present the pros and cons of passive physical therapy modalities, on the basis of the existing body of evidence, for the management of neck disorders namely whiplash-associated disorders and all other nonspecific neck disorders and complaints.

Findings: The existing body of evidence on effectiveness is extremely disappointing. Only a handful of studies have met minimal methodological standards in the field of physiotherapy, including medicine and surgery. Of all passive physical therapy modalities only mobilization/manipulation have shown some evidence of effectiveness.

Conclusions: The long list of passive physical therapy modalities must be drastically shortened. The impression that manual therapy and physiotherapy may be more efficacious than medicine in the management of neck disorders may be explained by the patient's desire for a more "holistic approach" which includes personal and physical contact. The cons of passive modalities are that they may lead to patient's passivity, inactivity and disability behavior. The

Alain-Y. Bélanger, BSc, MSc, PhD, PT, is Professor, Department of Physiotherapy, Faculty of Medicine, Laval University, Ste-Foy, P.Q., Canada, G1K 7P4.

[Haworth co-indexing entry note]: "The Pros and Cons of Passive Physical Therapy Modalities for Neck Disorders." Bélanger, Alain-Y. Co-published simultaneously in *Journal of Musculoskeletal Pain* [The Haworth Medical Press, an imprint of The Haworth Press, Inc.] Vol. 4, No. 4, 1996, pp. 125-134; and: *Musculoskeletal Pain Emanating from the Head and Neck: Current Concepts in Diagnosis, Management and Cost Containment* [ed: Murray E. Allen] The Haworth Medical Press, an imprint of The Haworth Press, Inc., 1996, pp. 125-134. Single or multiple copies of this article are available from The Haworth Document Delivery Service [1-800-342-9678, 9:00 a.m. - 5:00 p.m. [EST]. E-mail address: getinfo@haworth.com].

pros are that they provide a "unique occasion" to reassure the patient and to remind him/her about the necessity of keeping active and staying at work as long as it does not further "harm" the neck condition. *[Article copies available from The Haworth Document Delivery Service: 1-800-342-9678. E-mail address: getinfo@haworth.com]*

KEYWORDS. Whiplash, neck disorders, physical therapy, modalities

INTRODUCTION

High quality per cost health care is today's goal of government policy makers, third party payers and health consumers. All of them increasingly require documentation of effectiveness. For the benefit of health care and consumers there is now a growing body of documentation to suggest that the delivery system of health services will slowly, but inevitably, move from yesterday's "experience-based" to tomorrow's "evidence-based" practice (1). For example the recent literature on the management of soft-tissue injuries, namely back and neck disorders, represents a key example of this new shift from "experience" to "evidence-based" practice (2,3,4).

Physiotherapy [PT] is an important complement to medicine. The demand for PT is still increasing with the desire for well-being and mobility and with the expanding wish for innocuous alternatives to drugs and surgery for soft-tissue injuries. Patients with neck complaints are often treated by physicians and physiotherapists. Referral to physiotherapists is an option that is frequently used by general practitioners [GPs] and occasionally by medical specialists. In managing cases of neck complaints and disorders, physiotherapists often rely on the application of passive modalities. The purpose of this paper is to present the pros and cons of passive physical therapy modalities, on the basis of the existing body of evidence, for the management of neck disorders namely whiplash-associated disorders and all other nonspecific neck disorders.

EVIDENCE OF EFFECTIVENESS

We define as "passive" a physical therapy modality which does not require the patient to actively participate by either exerting a muscle contraction or performing a presumed therapeutic task while receiving the modality. Table 1 provides a summary of passive physical therapy modali-

TABLE 1. Evidence of Effectiveness of Passive Physical Therapy Modalities for Whiplash Associated Disorder.

Modalities	Summary of evidence
– Mobilization	• Five randomized controlled trials [RCTs] acceptable–used as an adjunct to strategies that promote activation. In combination with activating interventions, they appear to be beneficial in the short term, but long-term benefit has to be established. Brodin 1984; Brodin 1985; McKinney 1989; McKinney et al. 1989; Mealy et al. 1986
– Manipulation	• Only one acceptable study–a single manipulation compared to a single mobilization produced equivalent immediate [less than 5 minutes] improvements in pain and in range of motion. Because manipulation is a common treatment in WAD, its value must be established in RCTs. Cassidy et al. 1992
– Traction	• Only one acceptable study. No clinically or statistically significant differences in outcome between any of the traction types and the control treatment. Zybergold and Piper 1985
– Stretch and spray	• No studies were found.
– Transcutaneous nerve stimulation	• No acceptable studies were found.
– Electrical stimulation	• No accepted studies were found.
– Ultrasound	• No accepted studies were found.
– Laser, short-wave diathermy, heat, ice and massage	• No acceptable studies regarding the independent effect of any of these modalities.

ties which have been recently assessed for evidence of effectiveness by the Quebec Task Force [QTF] on whiplash-associated disorders [WAD] (4,5,6,7,8,9,10,11). Table 2 summarizes the results of a computer aided search of random control trials [RCTs] by Koes et al. (12,13,14,15,16), on the effectiveness of mobilization and manipulation for nonspecific neck disorders. Table 3 summarized the results of two studies by Koes et al. (17,18) on the effectiveness of manual therapy, physiotherapy, placebo therapy and medicine/general practitioner [GP] therapy for the treatment of nonspecific neck and back complaints, up to a one-year follow up, in 256 patients.

DISCUSSION AND CONCLUSION

Despite their exhaustive literature search, both the QTF (4) and Koes et al. (12) were disappointed by the studies evaluating the common therapeutic intervention or modalities for WAD and other nonspecific neck disorders. The bottom line is that existing studies are scientifically flawed and only a few have met minimum methodological research standards (4,12).

Reality Check

Over the past few years the use of passive physical modalities for neck and back disorders have been under the microscope of the medical and scientific communities and on the agenda of policy makers who are seeking high quality/low cost health care. To be more precise physiotherapy interventions, as opposed to medical and surgical interventions, have been seriously questioned on the critical issue of therapeutic effectiveness for neck and back disorders. Still today a large majority of patients, clinicians and policy makers are under the impression that medical and surgical interventions for neck disorders have been proven effective while physiotherapy interventions are still lacking proof of effectiveness. Does the body of evidence on effectiveness support this impression?

On the basis of the work done by the QTF (4) and Koes et al. (12) the evidence seems to support an impression that some PT interventions may be more efficacious for neck disorders than some medical or surgical interventions. While the QTF (4) on WAD, as shown in Table 1, was able to find seven articles on the effectiveness of passive physical modalities such as mobilization and manipulation, they were unable to find studies on the benefit of medical/drug interventions such as narcotic analgesics or psychopharmacologic therapeutics. Only two studies on nonsteroidal anti-

TABLE 2. Evidence of Effectiveness of Mobilization and Manipulation for Nonspecific Neck Disorders, after Koes et al. (12).

- Computer aided search found 5 randomized controlled trials
- Score of quality method—maximum of 100

Results:			
Sloop et al. (13)	50	Negative	Chronic neck pain
Nordemar et al. (14)	43	Negative	Acute neck pain
Brodin (15)	39	Positive	Acute plus chronic neck pain
Howe et al. (16)	29	Positive	Acute plus chronic neck pain

Positive: Better than the control treatment.

Negative: Worse than or equally effective as control treatment.

129

TABLE 3. Effectiveness of Manual Therapy, Physiotherapy, Placebo Therapy and Medicine-General Practitioner [GP] for the Treatment of Nonspecific Neck and Back Complaints up to a One-Year Followup, see Koes et al. (17).

	Manual therapy	Physiotherapy	Placebo therapy	Medicine/GP	All subjects
• No. of subjects	65	66	64	61	256
• No. of neck patients	13	21	14	16	64
• No. of treatments for all patients	5.4	14.7	11.1	1	—
• Duration of treatments [weeks] for all the patients	8.9	7.8	5.8	1	—

• **Caution:** No distinction was made by the authors between the neck, back and neck-back group of patients

• **Conclusions:**
  • More favorable outcome for treatment with manual therapy or physiotherapy vs. treatment by medicine/GP
  • Placebo therapy showed better results than treatment by medicine/GP
  • No difference in effectiveness between manual therapy and physiotherapy for all outcome measures at all follow up measurements. However the number of treatments [visits] was three times less for the manual therapy group [5.4 vs. 14.7] versus physiotherapy
  • Improvement of the main complaint in the manual therapy and physical therapy was consistently better than in the placebo group although the difference was not statistically significant at the 5% level.
  • Because patients responded remarkably well in the placebo therapy suggests the importance of the nonspecific effects of a referral. This is further supported by the fact that the placebo therapy group, who received approximately 11 sessions or treatment, showed better results than the treatment group by the GP, who had only one visit or treatment.

• **Bottom line:**
  • The possibility that "extra-attention" could produce improvement should be considered in the approach and treatment of patients with neck and back complaints.
  • After 12 months follow up both manipulative therapy and physiotherapy seem to be more effective than treatment by the general practitioner or placebo treatment in patients with persistent back and neck pain.

inflammatory drugs, combined with analgesics and other treatment modalities, were found by the QTF (4). Furthermore, the QTF was unable to find acceptable surgical studies of disk surgery–nerve block–rhizolisis–epidural or intrathecal steroid injections for the management of WAD. To further support the impression that PT interventions may be more efficacious than the traditional medical approach for nonspecific neck disorders, Koes et al. (17,18) found proof of effectiveness of physiotherapy/manual therapy over placebo therapy and medical/GP therapy.

What's Behind This Impression of Effectiveness?

It has been stated that "impressions are often misleading"! Well, in the case of management of neck and back disorders this dictum may be a truism! In fact a close look at the body of evidence not only demonstrated a profound lack of effectiveness across all professions, but also showed the failure of the common approaches by physiotherapists, physicians and surgeons. The blanket prescriptions of inactivity, drugs and passive physical therapy interventions has dominated the therapeutic approach, but has failed to show any benefit.

It is clear from the existing body of evidence that the long list of passive modalities must be drastically shortened. The use of many modalities, such as ultrasound and laser, can only be justified if they are part of a well-designed clinical trial where a placebo treatment is introduced, and so far they have failed.

The Pros and Cons of Passive Physical Therapy Modalities

The pros and cons are summarized in Table 4. The serial and prolonged application of passive modalities lacks any proof of effectiveness. It also leads the patient into adopting a passive role and reinforces inactivity and disability behavior. How can one argue that a judicious application of passive modalities may be necessary in the management of neck disorders? A possible answer may be found in Koes et al. (17,18) studies which found PT, manual therapy and even placebo therapy to be more efficacious than the medical/GP treatment. That placebo therapy was more effective than the medical/GP therapy strongly suggests the importance of a more "holistic approach" to the management of neck and back disorders and complaints, or that iatrogenic issues are invoked by some forms of treatment. A visit or two to a medical practitioner, followed by going home to wait while taking drugs and resting, may not be the solution to the management of neck pain.

TABLE 4. The Pros and Cons of Passive Physical Therapy Modalities for Whiplash Associated Disorders and Other Nonspecific Neck Disorders.

Cons	Pros
• Reinforce patient's passive role as health consumer	• Meet the urgent need patients have to establish prompt and personalized physical mobilization/manipulation and verbal contacts with a qualified health practitioner
• Promote the visible role clinicians want to play as "biological healers"	• Meet the need for a more "holistic approach"—clinicians treat an individual, not only his/her neck
• Promote patient's inactivity	• Allow the clinician to offer this "extra-attention," which may be associated with placebo therapy, to his/her patient
• Promote patient's awareness of pain	• Allow the clinician the time to:
• Reinforce disability behavior	• reassure the patient—decrease anxiety
• Reinforce the "biological" importance of neck disorders	• instruct as to what to do and not to do in relation to work, leisure and activities of daily living
• Promote the "medicalization of neck disorders"	• remind the patient to keep active
	• remind the patient to stay at work as long as it does not "harm" the condition further

Why is it that manual therapy was slightly better than PT which was slightly better than placebo therapy for non-specific neck complaints (17,18)? The answer may be the personal contact between the patient and a qualified health practitioner–in this case a physiotherapist. Another important factor is the number of visits or treatments. Clearly, more than one visit is necessary but the number should be kept low in keeping with the evidence which demonstrates only a short-term effect from mobilization or manipulation on neck complaints (4). However, the optimum number of visits by whatever profession has not been established.

It is here proposed that if passive physiotherapy modalities are used, that this "therapy time" be used to deliver reassurance, allay fears, instruct on activities of daily living and mobilizing activities, and to insure on continued work or early return to work, which is the penultimate success of any therapy.

REFERENCES

1. Evidence-Based Medicine Working Group: Evidence-Based Medicine: A new approach to teaching the practice of medicine. JAMA 4: 2420-2425, 1992.

2. Spitzer WO, [with Bélanger AY et al.].: Scientific approach to the assessment and management of activity-related spinal disorders. Spine 12(7S): S1-S57, 1987.

3. Bigos S, Bowyer O, Braen G, et al.: Acute Low Back Problems in Adults: Clinical Practice Guideline #14. AHCPR Publication No 95-0642, Rockville, MD, 1994.

4. Spitzer WO, et al.: Scientific Monograph of the Quebec Task Force on Whiplash-Associated Disorders: Redefining "Whiplash" and its management. Spine Suppl 20: S1-S73, 1995.

5. Brodin H: Cervical pain and mobilization. Int J Rehab Res 7: 190-191, 1984.

6. Brodin H: Cervical pain and mobilization. J Man Med 2: 18-22, 1985.

7. McKinney JA: Early mobilization and outcome in acute sprains of the neck. BMJ 299: 1006-1008, 1989.

8. McKinney LA, Dornan JO, Ryan M: The role of physiotherapy in the management of acute neck sprains following road-traffic events. Arch Emerg Med 6: 27-33, 1989.

9. Mealy K, Brennan H, Fenelon GC: Early mobilization of acute whiplash injuries. BMJ 282: 656-657, 1986.

10. Cassidy JD, Lopes AA, Yong-Hing K: The immediate effect of manipulation versus mobilization on pain and range of motion in the cervical spine: A randomized controlled trial. J Man Physiol Ther 15: 570-575, 1992.

11. Zylbergold RS, Piper MC: Cervical spine disorders: A comparison of three types of traction. Spine 10: 867-871, 1985.

12. Koes BW, Assendelft WJJ, Van der Heijden GJMG, Bouter LM, Knips-child PG: Spinal manipulation and mobilization for back and neck pain: A blinded review. BMJ 303: 1278-1303, 1991.

13. Sloop PR, Smith DS, Goldenberg E, Doré C: Manipulation for chronic neck pain: A double blind controlled study. Spine 7: 32-35, 1982.

14. Nordemar R, Thorner C: Treatment of acute cervical pain: A comparative group study. Pain 10: 93-101, 1981.

15. Brodin H: Cervical pain and mobilization. Med Phys. 6: 67-72, 1983.

16. Howe DH, Newcome R: Manipulation of the cervical spine. JR Coll Gen Pract 33: 574-579, 1983.

17. Koes BW, Bouter LM, Van Mameren H, Essers AHM, Vertegen GMJR, Hofhuizen DM, Houben JP, Knipschild PG: The effectiveness of manual therapy, physiotherapy, and treatment by general practitioner for nonspecific back and neck complaints. Spine 17: 28-35, 1992.

18. Koes BW, Bouter LM, Van Mameren H, Essers AHM, Vertegen GMJR, Hofhuizen DM, Houben JP, Knipschild PG: Randomized clinical trial of manipu-lative therapy and physiotherapy for persistent back and neck complaints: Results of one year follow up. BMJ 304: 601-605, 1992.

Longitudinal Course of Behavioral and Physical Findings in Temporomandibular Disorders

Samuel F. Dworkin

SUMMARY. The widely accepted use of a bio-psycho-social model to conceptualize the etiology, maintenance and management of disease conditions, including musculoskeletal pain conditions, has demonstrable clinical implications. For chronic musculoskeletal conditions such as temporomandibular disorders [TMD], factors influencing the oft-found disparities between symptom report, clinical observation and responses to treatment are more likely to involve behavioral, cognitive and emotional processes than pathophysiologic processes. Analyses of longitudinal data from population based studies and clinical trials involving biobehavioral interventions for TMD with follow-up periods from one to five years, provide empirical support that concurrent consideration of physiologic and psychologic findings is indicated in clinical management decisions of both primary and tertiary health care providers. A model currently being developed is presented to explain the relationship between saliency of perceived physical versus psychological symptoms and choices made with regard to deciding to seek biomedical or psychiatric types of health care. *[Article copies available from The Haworth Document Delivery Service: 1-800-342-9678. E-mail address: getinfo@haworth.com]*

Samuel F. Dworkin, DDS, PhD, is Professor, Department of Oral Medicine, School of Dentistry, and Department of Psychiatry and Behavioral Sciences, School of Medicine, University of Washington, Seattle, WA 98195.

[Haworth co-indexing entry note]: "Longitudinal Course of Behavioral and Physical Findings in Temporomandibular Disorders." Dworkin, Samuel F. Co-published simultaneously in *Journal of Musculoskeletal Pain* [The Haworth Medical Press, an imprint of The Haworth Press, Inc.] Vol. 4, No. 4, 1996, pp. 135-144; and: *Musculoskeletal Pain Emanating from the Head and Neck: Current Concepts in Diagnosis, Management and Cost Containment* [ed: Murray E. Allen] The Haworth Medical Press, an imprint of The Haworth Press, Inc., 1996, pp. 135-144. Single or multiple copies of this article are available from The Haworth Document Delivery Service [1-800-342-9678, 9:00 a.m. - 5:00 p.m. [EST]. E-mail address: getinfo@haworth.com].

KEYWORDS. Temporomandibular, whiplash, chronic pain, psychological, behavior

INTRODUCTION

Biomedical care, in this case medical and dental treatment, is typically focused on the diagnosis and management of physical conditions and pathophysiologic processes. Yet, it is increasingly understood that emotionally distressed patients have more doctor visits, and more hospitalizations. Moreover, those with emotional distress visit doctors with what appears to be non-specific physical symptoms—fatigue, dizziness, and of special relevance are a number of common pain complaints, notably back, neck and head pain and pain related to temporomandibular disorders (1).

When taken together with the data of others, we find support for the notion that presentation of physical symptoms not associated with diagnosable organic disease is widespread, a common and potentially misunderstood problem in treatment settings, and perhaps for a significant minority of patients, indicative of a need to review how we presently dichotomize diagnoses into independent emotional and physical categories, for example, into depression versus TMD versus fibromyalgia versus chronic fatigue syndrome, etc. (2,3).

Longitudinal data comes from clinical examination of TMD clinic cases at baseline, 1, 3 and 5 year follow-up and from psychological scales of depression and somatization which are part of the SCL-90-R, a symptom checklist measure. We have normative values for these scales for the Northwestern United States, derived from large population based studies of Group Health Cooperative of Puget Sound [GHC] enrollees, who are also the source for many of our clinic cases (4). The GHC is a large [enrollees >350,000] health maintenance organization [HMO] in the Pacific Northwestern United States. In addition to the clinical physical findings and psychological assessment, data from the automated data records of GHC with regard to frequency of medical visits and patient report of TMD treatment sought have been examined.

CLINICAL FINDINGS

One aspect of psychological status which might influence clinical findings is "somatization," defined as the predisposition to identify non-specific bodily sensations as symptoms of disease or illness (5). We examined the relationship between high and low levels of somatization in our clinic cases–the top and bottom quartiles in this analysis, and related level of somatization to the number of masticatory and adjacent muscles tender to digital, or palpation examination, by a calibrated reliable TMD examiner [not the treating clinician]. In a separate series of TMD cases seen in 1986 and 1992, we observed that those in the highest quartile for somatization had from two to three times as many painful palpation sites–whether extra- or intra-oral muscles of mastication or clinically diagnostic palpation sites for the temporomandibular joint–as those in the lowest quartile of the distribution with regard to somatization scores (6). Thus, extremes of somatization scores were, in effect, highly predictive of the numbers of masticatory structures painful to diagnostic palpation.

In addition to determining muscles and joint sites tender to palpation, the assessment of mandibular range of motion is also one of the cardinal clinical signs entering into the differential diagnosis of TMD (7,8). Ambiguity exists regarding whether all components of these clinical findings are objective signs or subjective symptoms of TMD. The question is important because the major criteria for diagnosing TMD are perceived to be subjective, self-report symptoms. Reporting of such symptoms may be influenced by non-specific factors such as widespread presence of symptoms elsewhere in the body; therefore, emotional and behavioral factors become the major influences of pain perception and treatment seeking behavior. In effect, our current ability to differentially diagnose TMD from other conditions would be a function of psychological or psychosocial level of functioning. These factors would be a reflection of pathophysiologic processes detectable by objective measurement.

This problem of how to view clinical findings of TMD, as signs or symptoms, is well known to researchers and clinicians alike. It seems fair to say that diagnosis of TMD is considered, for the most part, a diagnosis of a symptom state, more specifically, a diagnosis of a pain symptom state. In a number of previous reports we, as well as others, have presented data demonstrating the usefulness of viewing TMD primarily as a chronic pain condition and have demonstrated that TMD shares many symptom-reporting and behavioral findings observed in the most common chronic pain conditions we know, such as headache and back pain (9-11).

Interaction with Patterns of Health Care Utilization. Somatization as a clinically relevant factor is more complex than merely asking for subjective reporting of non-specific physical symptoms. Its clinical relevance derives from how much treatment seeking certain patients may undertake in order to seek relief from these perceived physical symptoms, which again, are not dependable indicators of pathophysiology (12,13). So, we also examined treatment seeking patterns in relation to somatization levels as scored from the SCL-90 and related both the level of somatization and extent of treatment seeking behavior to critical parameters of TMD.

Turning to our initial longitudinal analyses, the initial data is limited to one-year follow-up of a sample of GHC clinic cases and includes automated data allowing us to assess total number of medical visits in the prior year. This treatment seeking data does not include TMD treatment visits, representing treatment visits for all medical reasons for these patients.

High and low somatization and number of medical visits were defined as representing the top 30% and bottom 30% in each category. The subjectively reported average pain intensity for the group as a whole, at baseline, was 39.7, derived from a 0-100 visual analogue score where 0 = no pain and 100 = the most unbearable pain imaginable.

Those who scored in the lowest 30% of somatization scores and were in the lowest 30% of users of health care had average baseline pain intensity of 29.1, while those at the high end on both parameters of somatization and health care visits yield average TMD pain intensity of 53.5. Of interest, self-report of many non-specific symptoms, by itself, was not as prognostic of future pain level as was the combination of self-reported symptoms and actual number of medical visits; for example, after one year, average pain levels dropped for all groups except those high in both somatization score and number of medical visits.

Turning to determination of muscle palpation sites, using the same high and low groupings of somatization score and numbers of medical visits, a similar pattern observed for subjective pain report was noted. Those lowest in both subjective report of non-specific physical symptoms and in treatment seeking behavior had, at baseline, the lowest number of muscle palpation sites, averaging 3.7, compared to a mean of 5.3 for the group as a whole, while those highest in both baseline categories reported an average of 6.4 masticatory muscles painful to palpation, using calibrated and reliable examiners and examination methods.

When muscle palpation sites were diagnostically evaluated using the same longitudinal analyses, the number of masticatory muscle sites tender to palpation significantly decreased on one-year follow-up for all combinations of high-low somatization and treatment seeking levels, except, again, for those high in both. Thus, baseline high levels of somatization and heightened treatment seeking behavior became associated, one year later with even more tender muscle sites than were diagnosed initially.

Pain intensity is universally acknowledged to be a subjective phenomenon. Diagnostically evaluating masticatory muscles depends on the report of pain. However, it has been shown that the pain response to a standarized diagnostic muscle palpation test is influenced by psychological status (8,14).

Seeking an objective diagnostic measure for TMD, we again examined the relationship between somatization score and treatment seeking behavior, but this time related those findings to measurement of maximally assisted vertical jaw opening, considered an objective test because, for the most part, since the dentist opens the patients mouth as much as possible, there is less room for subjective factors to influence the final measurement. And, indeed, when values for maximally assisted jaw opening were examined we found no baseline relationship with somatization score or number of medical visits. The mean maximum assisted opening for the group as a whole was 47.1 mm, which remained fairly constant, tending to increase [not statistically significant] after one year, for all the high and low groups being studied. Thus, when the longitudinal relationship between levels of somatization, treatment visits and the more objective diagnostic sign of maximum assisted jaw opening was examined, there was virtually no change observed from initial values recorded at baseline, indicating that psychological status, as assessed by somatization score and treatment seeking behavior, as assessed by total number of medical visits, seemed to have no influence on a clinical sign of TMD which does not, by definition, depend on the subjective.

Findings from Five-Year Follow-Up Studies. Extending these types of analyses to five-year longitudinal data for TMD clinic cases, which parenthetically, comprises a truly unique data set for this field, we were interested in depicting the relationship between longitudinal patterns of TMD pain and longitudinal course of selected TMD signs and symptoms.

For purposes of these preliminary analyses, we identified patients who, at the five-year follow-up, met the criteria for being pain-free, improved in amount of average pain by at least 50% from their baseline level of pain, and those whose pain remained constant or worsened, with regard to baseline values. After five-years, about half the patients were pain free and the remaining half about equally divided among those whose pain improved, worsened or remained constant.

We examined the relationship over five years among the four pain patterns we defined with their clinical signs and symptoms. Signs included number of TMJ sounds believed to be indicative of present or future joint or disc pathologies, and maximum vertical range of motion. Pain history was found to be unrelated to presence or development of increased number of signs; as a matter of fact a significant interaction, was observed indicating that those whose pain was constant at five years relative to baseline, had less TMJ sounds such as joint click, crepitus or grating on five year follow-up. The same [essentially non-meaningful] relationship was observed between course of pain over five years and maximum vertical range of jaw motion, another important sign of TMD—that is, maximum range of jaw motion stayed essentially constant or increased slightly over five years, whether pain remitted, improved, remained constant or worsened. As we moved towards assessment of clinical findings that invoke self-report of pain, greater variability emerges where patients are asked to open their mouth until pain is experienced. Those destined to be pain-free show a significantly greater pain-free range of motion compared to those whose pain remained constant, worsened or improved.

When the relationship between pain pattern and patterns of change in numbers of muscles tender to palpation were examined, the only significant finding was that those whose pain remained constant or worse maintained higher levels of tender muscles than those who were pain free. Those who improved in pain level were not significantly different either from those eventually pain-free or those who wound up with high levels of pain.

At this point we interpret this data to mean that self-reported patterns of pain, whether the pain goes away, remains constant, improves or worsens, is relatively independent of available objective clinical examination findings, while more subjectively involved clinical findings which invoke pain reporting [e.g., as when pain-free jaw opening is measured] are sometimes better related to overall average levels of ambient pain.

When the relationship between somatization and pain pattern was examined a very different picture of variability emerged. In general, pain pattern seemed better related to changes in somatization: those who wound up pain-free or improved reach population mean levels for somatization, while those whose pain over five years worsened or remained constant relative to baseline consistently showed significantly elevated levels of somatization, placing them well in the top quartile of the population scores for somatization.

Interestingly, the same pattern is not observed for depression, in that for all types of longitudinal pain patterns, SCL levels of depression tend to be at the population mean or below, after five years. The constant and worse groups show the same trend to maintain their initial levels of depression, but not significantly, as was true of somatization.

We next analyzed whether or not extent and timing of TMD treatment was related to changes in these same objective and subjective clinical variables. We identified four patterns of treatment: 1. treatment received prior to baseline only; 2. treatment received in every follow-up interval; 3. no TMD treatment ever received; 4. other. About 60% of the patients had received treatment prior to coming to our clinic and entering the study, and the remaining 40% was almost equally divided among those defined as receiving maximum treatment [having received prior treatment and treatment during every follow-up interval for the course of our five-year study], those who received no treatment at all and those who received treatment only in the course of the study, but had not received TMD treatment prior to being enrolled in our five year study.

Briefly summarizing the relationship over time between amount of TMD treatment received and changes in number of joint sounds, vertical range of motion, somatization and depression, we observed that the amount of treatment sought was not related to changes in any of these variables. At five years all groups were equivalent on the respective variables, except for somatization, which achieved normative values only for the group that received no treatment during the five-year study period. The minimal interpretation at this stage seems to be that the amount of treatment is not importantly related to clinical signs and symptoms, but much more analysis is needed to inquire into types of treatment received before this conclusion can be confirmed.

Somatization and Depression. The final data demonstrated a relationship in TMD clinic cases between depression and somatization, that is, those reporting the highest number of non-specific physical symptoms were also those found to hold significantly elevated depression scores. Do these people have three illnesses: depression, somatization disorder, and TMD? We know from our previous reports that those individuals with multiple pain complaints are at high risk for meeting criteria for major depression as assessed by the SCL-90 (1).

The presence of a somatization process is associated with the predisposition to hold a biomedical model of disease, that is, the view that all symptoms have a physical or pathophysiologic basis, exclusively, as opposed to a biopsychosocial model of illness, where the view is that symptoms may represent adaptive or maladaptive coping with physical and or mental processes and presented data to support this view that those predisposed towards somatization hold predominately a biomedical explanation for their symptoms (15).

Goldberg (16), widely known for his psychiatric epidemiology studies of mental disorders in primary care, has identified the frequency with which those disorders are seen in primary care. Thus, from the general population, of 590 new primary care medical consultations in Manchester, England, approximately 67% were not associated with any mental disorder while about 20% met his criteria for somatization. These criteria included treatment seeking for somatic symptoms attributed to a physical disease, but which cannot be confirmed medically, and the presence of anxiety or depression as a mental disorder. Of the psychiatric cases, 57% presenting to primary care physicians for management of somatic symptoms met criteria for somatization. Thus, Goldberg views somatization as one of the common mental disorders and the physical symptoms presented in those cases are to be interpreted as part of the mental disorder. According to Goldberg, patients who complain of somatic symptoms in general medical settings, in the absence of a physical cause, and who do not consider themselves psychologically ill can be described as somatizers, and they constitute the commonest kind of new psychological disorder.

Simon (17) has examined data from Wave I of the National Institute of Mental Health Epidemiologic Catchment Area [NIMHECA] study to determine how non-specific somatic symptoms and other psychiatric disorders relate to use of health care. Simon's data indicated that somatization was linked to general medical visits but not to mental health visits. Major depression, while more heavily involving mental health services, still was associated with high numbers of general medical visits, especially for women, that is, distressed individuals present their physical symptoms to medical settings, whether their distress is limited to somatization concerns or includes such psychiatric disorders as major depression. Katon (12) has suggested that somatization be conceptualized as a spectrum of severity. While the entire range is of concern to both medical and mental health clinicians and researchers, the more severe end of the spectrum [somatization associated with the presentation of as many as 11-14 non-specific physical symptoms] occurs infrequently. Thus, the lower-middle ranges of the somatization spectrum [involving the presentation of four-five non-specific physical symptoms] represents the more common challenge to health care providers.

Developing an Explanatory Model. We have attempted to elaborate an explanatory model (18) reflective of our understanding of the relationship between perceiving symptoms and seeking treatment. The schema reflects our understanding that all symptoms, including physical symptoms such as pain, arise from the interaction of multiple factors–genetic, developmental, and environmental as they encounter precipitating events. When the events are negative, or interpreted as negative, the resolution of this dynamic process is distress–a dynamic, dysphoric organismic state which is noxious or aversive and from which relief is sought. Specifically, relief is sought from the experience of negative or aversive symptoms and the form of the relief can include attempts to cope which are adaptive or maladaptive. Beginning with Engel's (19) introduction of the biopsychosocial model and followed by Mechanic's (20) distinction between disease and illness and the current work of Kleinman (21) with explanatory models for illness, we now understand that the type of health care that is included in response to these physical and psychological symptoms will be influenced by explanatory models, or belief systems the patient holds about the cause, exacerbation, and available sources of relief for their problem.

Patients detecting and reporting physical symptoms, such as pain which interferes with physical function and which they attribute to physical disease will seek out treatment from the biomedical components of the health care system as opposed to seeking psychiatric or psychologically based therapies [e.g., one of the many currently available forms of psychotherapy].

CONCLUSION

Focusing on TMD as a chronic pain condition, published and preliminary data has been presented which relate to the potential for psychological factors to influence clinical decision-making and the diagnosis of TMD. The diagnosis of TMD requires subjective self-report of clinical symptoms, including the presence of pain, assessment of limitations in jaw movement dependent on the subjects report of pain and assessment of muscles tender to palpation, again as determined by subjective pain report in response to a calibrated muscle palpation diagnostic test.

We have attempted to demonstrate that psychological status, for present purposes limiting data to somatization, influence both the subjective perception of pain intensity reported and the number of muscles reported as painful to diagnostic palpation test. We have also discussed how somatization may influence the extent of treatment seeking in non-specific ways. We conclude that attempts to arrive at clinical diagnoses of TMD may be confounded for patients who reveal predispositions towards somatization by the report of numerous non-specific physical symptoms which may extend to the predisposition to heightened reports of pain and painful muscles. The role of somatization as factor influencing treatment outcome has also been reported by McCreary (13), who concludes that failure to recognize and manage somatization in TMD patients is associated with poor treatment outcomes.

REFERENCES

1. Dworkin SF, Von Korff MR, LeResche L: Multiple pains and psychiatric disturbance: An epidemiologic investigation. Arch Gen Psychiatry 47:239-244, 1990.

2. Sullivan M: The path between distress and somatic symptoms. Am Pain Society J 2:141-149, 1993.

3. Wolfe F, Cathey MA: The epidemiology of tender points: A prospective study of 1520 patients. J Rheumatol 12:1164-1168, 1985.

4. Von Korff M, Dworkin SF, LeResche L, et al.: An epidemiologic comparison of pain complaints. Pain 32:173-183, 1988.

5. Katon W: Somatization in primary care. J Fam Pract 21[4]:257-258, 1985.

6. Wilson L, Dworkin SF, Whitney C, et al.: Somatization and pain dispersion in chronic temporomandibular pain. Pain 57:55-61, 1994.

7. American Dental Association: The President's conference on the dentist-patient relationship and the management of fear, anxiety and pain. Chicago, American Dental Association, 1983.

8. Dworkin SF, LeResche L: Research diagnostic criteria for temporomandibular disorders. J Craniomandib Disord Facial Oral Pain 6:301-355, 1992.

9. Dworkin SF: Personal and societal impact of orofacial pain. In Fricton JR, Dubner RB [eds]: Orofacial pain and temporomandibular disorders. New York, Raven Press, 1995, 15-32.

10. Rudy TE, Turk DC, Zaki HS, et al.: An empirical taxometric alternative to traditional classification of temporomandibular disorders. Pain 36:311-320, 1989.

11. Rugh JD, Woods BJ, Dahlstrom L: Temporomandibular disorders: Assessment of psychosocial factors. Adv Dent Res 7:127-136, 1993.

12. Katon W, Lin E, Von Korff M, et al.: Somatization: A spectrum of severity. Am J Psychiatry 148:34-40, 1991.

13. McCreary CP, Clark GT, Oakley ME, et al.: Predicting response to treatment for temporomandibular disorders. J Craniomandib Disord Facial Oral Pain 6[3]:161-169, 1992.

14. Fricton JR, Kroening RJ, Hathaway KM: TMJ and craniofacial pain: diagnosis and management. St. Louis, Ishiyaku EuroAmerica, 1987.

15. Massoth DL, Dworkin SF: Patient explanatory models for temporomandibular disorders [TMD]. J Dent Res 72[IADR Abstracts]:1993 [Abstract].

16. Goldberg D, Huxley P: Common mental disorders: A bio-social model. London, Tavistock/Routledge, 1992.

17. Simon GE: Somatization and psychiatric disorders. In Kirmayer LJ, Robbins JM [eds]: Progress in psychiatry: No. 31. Current concepts of somatization: Research and clinical perspectives. Vol 31. Washington DC, American Psychiatric Press, Inc. 1993, 37-61.

18. Dworkin SF, Wilson L, Massoth DL: Somatizing as a risk factor for chronic pain. In Grzesiak RC, Ciccone DS [eds]: Psychologic vulnerability to chronic pain. In press, 1993.

19. Engel G: The need for a new medical model: A challenge for biomedicine. Science 196:129-136, 1977.

20. Mechanic D: Social psychologic factors affecting the presentation of bodily complaints. N Engl J Med 286[21]:1132-1139, 1972.

21. Kleinman A: The Illness Narratives: Suffering, healing and the human condition. New York, Basic Books, Inc. 1988.

Psychological Aspects
of Chronic Pain and Disability

Dennis C. Turk

SUMMARY. Traditional views of pain as either directly associated with physical pathology or psychologically based [psychogenic or motivational] have proven to be inadequate. A range of psychological variables and concepts have been shown to play important roles in pain perception, maintenance and exacerbation of pain, disability, and response to treatment. The role of operant conditioning [learning] and cognitive factors [i.e., beliefs, perceptions of control, coping strategies] on the maintenance and exacerbation of pain and disability are reviewed. Particular attention is given to the effects of psychological factors on behavioral responses and physiological activity associated with pain. It is suggested that rather than viewing the pain experience as either organically-based or psychologically-based that both of these factors need to be viewed as contributors to the perception and response to pain. *[Article copies available from The Haworth Document Delivery Service: 1-800-342-9678. E-mail address: getinfo@haworth.com]*

Dennis C. Turk, PhD, is Professor of Psychiatry, Anesthesiology and Behavioral Science and Director, Pain Evaluation and Treatment Institute, University of Pittsburg Medical Center.

Address correspondence to: Dennis C. Turk, PhD, Pain Evaluation and Treatment Institute, University of Pittsburgh School of Medicine, 4601 Baum Boulevard, Pittsburgh, PA 15213.

[Haworth co-indexing entry note]: "Psychological Aspects of Chronic Pain and Disability." Turk, Dennis C. Co-published simultaneously in *Journal of Musculoskeletal Pain* [The Haworth Medical Press, an imprint of The Haworth Press, Inc.] Vol. 4, No. 4, 1996, pp. 145-153; and: *Musculoskeletal Pain Emanating from the Head and Neck: Current Concepts in Diagnosis, Management and Cost Containment* [ed: Murray E. Allen] The Haworth Medical Press, an imprint of The Haworth Press, Inc., 1996, pp. 145-153. Single or multiple copies of this article are available from The Haworth Document Delivery Service [1-800-342-9678, 9:00 a.m. - 5:00 p.m. [EST]. E-mail address: getinfo@haworth.com].

KEYWORDS. Patients' beliefs, cognitive-behavioral conceptualization, gate control model, motivation, operant conditioning, psychogenic model

INTRODUCTION

Chronic pain, by definition, extends over long periods of time. It is a demoralizing situation that confronts the individual not only with the stress created by organic factors and pain, but with a cascade of ongoing stressors that compromise all aspects of the life of the sufferer. Living with chronic pain requires considerable emotional resilience and tends to deplete one's emotional reserve, and taxes not only the individual but also the capacity of family, friends, coworkers, and employers to provide support.

UNDERSTANDING PERSISTENT PAIN AND DISABILITY ALTERNATIVE CONCEPTUALIZATIONS

Biomedical Model

The traditional biomedical view of pain dates back several hundred years and is based on a simple linear view that assumes a close correspondence between a biological state and symptom perception. From the traditional view, the extent of pain severity is presumed to be directly proportionate to the amount of tissue damage. Consequently, tissue damage is the sole cause for the report of pain and a specific physically-based treatment should be provided to alleviate the symptoms. The adequacy of this model has been challenged by clinical observation as well as research.

Psychogenic Model

As is frequently the case in medicine, when physical explanations prove inadequate to explain symptoms, psychological alternatives are invoked. If the pain reported is disproportionate to objectively determined physical pathology or if the complaint is recalcitrant to "appropriate" treatment, then it is assumed that psychological factors must be involved, even if not causal.

The psychogenic view is posed as an alternative to purely physiological models. Put quite simply, dichotomous reasoning is invoked. If the patient's report of pain occurs in the absence of or is "disproportionate" to objective physical pathology, ipso facto, the pain reports have a psychological basis.

Motivational View

A variation of the dichotomous organic versus psychogenic view is a conceptualization that is ascribed to by many third-party payers. This view suggests that if there is insufficient physical pathology to justify the report of pain, the complaint is invalid, the result of symptom exaggeration or outright malingering. The assumption is that reports of pain without adequate biomedical evidence are motivated exclusively by financial gain. There are, however, no studies that have demonstrated dramatic improvement in pain reports subsequent to receiving disability awards.

Operant Conditioning Model

Fordyce (1) proposed an alternative to the views outlined above. His operant conditioning model suggests that when an individual is exposed to a stimulus that causes tissue damage, the immediate response is withdrawal and attempts to escape from noxious sensations. This may be accomplished by avoidance of activity believed to cause or exacerbate pain, help-seeking to reduce symptoms, and so forth. These behaviors are observable, capable of eliciting a response from an observer, and; consequently, subject to the principles of operant conditioning. According to the operant conditioning model, positive reinforcement such as attention by avoidance of undesirable or feared activities may serve to maintain the pain behaviors even in the absence of noxious sensory input. In this way, respondent behaviors that occur following an acute injury may be maintained by reinforcement after any tissue damage has resolved.

The operant conditioning model does not concern itself with the initial cause or report of pain. Rather it considers pain an internal subjective experience that may be maintained even after an initial physical cause of pain has resolved. The operant conditioning model focuses on overt manifestations of pain and suffering—"pain behaviors"—such as limping, moaning and avoiding activity. Emphasis is placed on the communicative function of these behaviors and the responses they elicit from others.

A particularly important feature of conditioning models of pain is pain avoidance. Fordyce, Shelton, and Dundore (2) hypothesized that avoidance behavior does not necessarily require intermittent sensory stimulation from the site of bodily damage, environmental reinforcement, or successful avoidance of aversive social activity to account for the maintenance of protective movements. They suggested that protective behaviors could be maintained by anticipation of aversive consequences based on prior learning since on-occurrence of pain is a powerful reinforcer.

The operant principal of stimulus generalization is also important as patients may come to avoid more and more activities that they believe are similar to those that previously produced pain. Reduction of activity leads to greater physical deconditioning, more activities eliciting pain, and consequently even greater disability.

Multidimensional Models of Persistent Pain and Disability

The variability of patient responses to nociceptive stimuli and treatment is somewhat more understandable when we consider that pain is a personal experience influenced by attention, anxiety, prior learning, the meaning of the situation, other physiological and environmental factors, as well as physical pathology. Biomedical factors, in the majority of cases, appear to instigate the initial report of pain. Overtime, however, psychosocial and behavioral factors may serve to maintain and exacerbate levels of pain, influence adjustment and disability. Following from this view, pain that persists over time should not be viewed as either solely physical or psychological, rather the experience of pain is maintained by and interdependent set of biomedical, psychosocial, and behavioral factors. Two complementary models have been proposed that integrate organic and psychological contributors to pain–the gate control model and cognitive-behavioral conceptualization.

Gate Control Model

Melzack and his colleagues (3,4) proposed the gate control theory of pain that emphasized the modulation of pain by peripheral as well as central nervous system processes. This model provided a physiological basis for the role of psychological factors in chronic pain. Melzack and Casey (3) differentiated three systems related to the processing of nociceptive stimulation–motivational-affective, cognitive-evaluative, and sensory-discriminative–all thought to contribute to the subjective experience of pain. The gate control model has had a substantial impact on basic research and in generating a wide range of treatment modalities.

Cognitive-Behavioral Conceptualization

If one accepts that chronic pain is a complex, subjective phenomenon that is uniquely experienced by each individual; then knowledge about idiosyncratic beliefs, appraisals, and coping repertoires become critical for optimal treatment planning and for accurately evaluating treatment outcome.

Biomedical factors that may have initiated the original report of pain play less and less of a role in disability over time, although secondary problems associated with deconditioning may exacerbate and serve to maintain the problem. Inactivity leads to increased focus on and preoccupation with the body and pain, and these cognitive-attentional changes increase the likelihood of misinterpreting physiological processes, overemphasis on symptoms, and the perception of oneself as being disabled. Reduction of activity, fear of re-injury, pain, loss of compensation, and an environment that, perhaps, unwittingly supports the "pain patient role" can impede alleviation of pain, successful rehabilitation, and reduction of disability.

Patients' beliefs, appraisals, and expectations about their pain, their ability to cope, their social supports, their disorder, the medicolegal system, the health care system, and their employers are all important as they may facilitate or disrupt the patient's sense of control and ability to manage pain. These factors also influence patients' investment in treatment, acceptance of responsibility for self-care [e.g., performance of exercises], perceptions of disability, expectancies for treatment, acceptance of treatment rationale, and adherence to treatment recommendations (5,6).

From the cognitive-behavioral perspective, people with chronic pain are viewed as active processors of information. They may hold expectations about their own ability and responsibility to exert any control over their pain. Moveover, they often view themselves as helpless. The specific thoughts and feelings that patients experienced prior to exacerbations of pain, during an exacerbation or intense episode of pain, as well as following a pain episode can greatly influence the experience of pain and subsequent pain episodes.

Negative, maladaptive appraisals about their condition, situation, and their personal efficacy in controlling their pain and problems associated with pain serve to reinforce the experience of demoralization, inactivity, and the overreaction to nociceptive stimulation. The methods patients use to control their emotional arousal and symptoms have been shown to be important predictors of both cognitive and behavioral responses (7). These cognitive appraisals influence behavior, leading to reduced effort, reduced perseverance in the face of difficulty, reduced activity, and increased psychological distress.

Cognitive interpretations also will affect how patients present symptoms to significant others, including health care providers and employers. The cognitive-behavioral perspective integrates the operant conditioning emphasis on external reinforcement and respondent view of learned fear and avoidance with the emphasis on patients' beliefs, attitudes, and expectancies.

Empirical studies have supported the important role of cognitive variables in the maintenance and exacerbation of pain. Thoughts about the controllability of pain, attributions about one's own ability to use specific pain coping responses, expectations concerning the possible outcomes of various coping efforts, and common erroneous beliefs about pain and disability have been shown to affect patients' behaviors and mood and thus, indirectly, the experience of pain. They have also been shown to have a direct affect on physiological processes associated with nociception.

Indirect Effect of Psychological Factors on Pain Experience and Disability

A person's cognitions [beliefs, appraisals, expectancies] regarding the consequences of an event and his or her ability to cope with these consequences, are hypothesized to impact functioning in two ways. They may have a direct influence on mood and an indirect one through their impact on coping efforts.

Psychological factors may act indirectly on pain and disability by reducing physical activity, and, consequently reducing muscle flexibility, strength, tone, and endurance. Fear of re-injury, fear of loss of disability compensation, and job dissatisfaction can also influence return to work.

Specific beliefs may lead to maladaptive coping, increased suffering and greater disability. Patients who believe their pain is likely to persist may be quite passive in their coping efforts and fail to make use of cognitive strategies or behavioral strategies to cope with pain. Patients who consider their pain to be an unexplainable mystery, may negatively evaluate their own abilities to control or decrease pain. They have been shown to be less likely to rate their coping strategies as effective in controlling and decreasing pain (8).

The persistence of avoidance of specific activities will reduce disconfirmations that would be followed by performance of specific behaviors (9). Insofar as pain-avoidance succeeds in preserving the over-predictions of pain and possible injury from repeated disconfirmation, they will continue unchanged. By contrast, engaging in behavior that produces significantly less pain than the patient expected will be followed by adjustments in subsequent predictions, and willingness to engage in previously feared and avoided activities.

Chronic pain patients tend to believe that they have limited ability to exert control over their pain. Such negative, maladaptive appraisals about the situation and personal efficacy may reinforce the experience of demoralization, inactivity, and over-reaction to nociceptive stimulation commonly observed in chronic pain patients (10). Beliefs that disability is a necessary consequence of pain, that activity despite pain is dangerous, and that pain is an acceptable excuse for neglecting responsibilities are likely to contribute to even greater disability.

Several investigators have suggested that a common set of cognitive errors will effect perceptions of pain and disability (7,11). A cognitive error may be defined as a negatively distorted belief about oneself or one's situation. Specific cognitive errors and distortions have been linked consistently to depression (11), self-reported pain severity (7), and disability (7) in chronic pain patients.

Self-regulation of pain and its impact depends upon the individual's specific ways of dealing with pain, adjusting to pain, and reducing or minimizing pain and distress caused by pain, therefore, their coping strategies. Coping is assumed to be manifested by spontaneously employed purposeful and intentional acts. Behavioral coping strategies include rest, medication, and use of relaxation. Cognitive coping strategies include various means of distracting oneself from pain, reassuring oneself that the pain will diminish, seeking information, and problem solving. Coping strategies are thought to act to alter both the perception of intensity of pain and one's ability to manage or tolerate pain and to continue everyday activities.

Not all coping strategies are adaptive. It seems likely that different strategies will be more effective than others for some individuals at some specific times but not necessarily for all individuals all of the time (12).

Direct Effect of Psychological Factors on Physiology

Several studies have suggested that psychological factors may have a direct effect of physiological parameters associated more directly with the production or exacerbation of nociception. Cognitive interpretations and affective arousal may have a direct effect on a patient's physiology specifically associated with nociception by increasing autonomic sympathetic nervous system arousal (13), endogenous opioid [endorphins] production (14), elevated levels of muscle tension (15).

Circumstances that are appraised as potentially threatening to safety or comfort are likely to generate strong physiological reactions. For example, Flor et al. (15) demonstrated that discussing stressful events and pain produced elevated levels of electromyographic [EMG] activity localized to the site of back pain patients' pain.

Bandura and his colleagues (14) directly examined the role of central opioid activity in cognitive control of pain. They provided training where subjects received instructions and practice in using different cognitive strategies for alleviating pain. They demonstrated that a. perceptions of control increased with cognitive training; b. perceptions of control predicted pain tolerance; and c. that naloxone blocked the effects of the cognitive coping strategies. The latter result implicates the direct effects of thoughts on the endogenous opioid system.

CONCLUSIONS

The studies reviewed above provide a good deal of support for the role of psychological factors in maintenance and exacerbation of chronic pain and disability. A large number of psychological variables have been demonstrated to have both an indirect effect and direct effect on pain and disability.

Patients all come to treatment with diverse sets of attitudes, beliefs, expectancies, and prior leaning histories. What the research reviewed above suggests is the importance of addressing these psychological factors as they are likely to influence how patients present themselves and respond to treatments offered. Viewing all patients with the same medical diagnosis as similar is likely to prove unsatisfactory. It would seem prudent to a. attempt to identify pain patients' idiosyncratic beliefs, b. address those beliefs that are inaccurate and potentially maladaptive, and c. to match coping strategies with patients individual differences. Understanding and successfully treating chronic pain patients and thereby reducing disability will require attention not only to the organic basis of the symptoms but to the cognitive and affectives responses of patients to noxious stimuli and their plight.

REFERENCES

1. Fordyce WE: Behavioral Methods for Chronic Pain and Illness. Mosby, St. Louis, 1976.

2. Fordyce WE, Shelton J, Dundore D: The modification of avoidance learning pain behaviors. J Behav Med 4: 405-414, 1982.

3. Melzack R, Casey KL: Sensory, motivational and central control determinants of pain: A new conceptual model. In D Kenshalo [ed.] The Skin Senses. 423-443, Thomas, Springfield, 1968.

4. Melzack R, Wall PD: Pain mechanisms: A new theory. Science 50: 971-979, 1965.

5. Slater MA, Hall HF, Atkinson JH, Garfin SR: Pain and impairment beliefs in chronic low back pain: Validation of the Pain and Impairment Relationship Scale [PAIRS]. Pain 44: 51-56, 1991.

6. Turk DC, Rudy TE: Persistent pain and the injured worker: Integrating biomedical, psychosocial, and behavioral factors. J Occupat Rehabil 1: 159-179, 1991.

7. Flor H, Turk DC: Chronic back pain and rheumatoid arthritis: Predicting pain and disability from cognitive variables. J Behav Med 11: 251-265, 1988.

8. Williams DA, Keefe FJ: Pain beliefs and the use of cognitive-behavioral coping strategies. Pain 46: 185-190, 1991.

9. Rachman S, Arntz A: The overprediction and underprediction of pain. Clin Psychol Rev 11: 339-356, 1991.

10. Biederman HJ, McGhie A, Monga TN, Shanks GL: Perceived and actual control in EMG treatment of back pain. Behav Res Ther 25: 137-147, 1987.

11. Gil KM, Williams DA, Keefe FJ, Beckham JC: The relationship of negative thoughts to pain and psychological distress. Behav Therap 21: 349-352, 1990.

12. Turk DC, Meichenbaum D, Genest M: Pain and Behavioral Medicine: A Cognitive-Behavioral Perspective. Guilford, New York, 1983.

13. Bandura A, Taylor CB, Williams SL, Mefford IN, Barchas JD: Catecholamine secretion as a function of perceived coping self-efficacy. J Consult Clin Psychol 53: 406-414, 1985.

14. Bandura A, O'Leary A, Taylor CB, Gauthier J, Gossard D: Perceived self-efficacy and pain control: Opioid and nonopioid mechanisms. J Personal Soc Psychol 53: 563-571, 1987.

15. Flor H, Turk DC, Birbaumer N: Assessment of stress-related responses in chronic back pain patients. J Consult Clin Psychol 53: 354-364, 1995.

Temporomandibular Pain-Dysfunction Syndrome: Evidence for Psychological Etiology?

Joseph J. Marbach

SUMMARY. Objective: To present evidence on the relation of psychological factors to the etiology and maintenance of the temporomandibular pain and dysfunction syndrome [TMPDS].

Findings and Conclusions: There is a lack of evidence that the etiology of TMPDS is psychological. However, psychological stress may play a role in the maintenance of pain through its capacity as a source of exacerbation. *[Article copies available from The Haworth Document Delivery Service: 1-800-342-9678. E-mail address: getinfo@haworth.com]*

INTRODUCTION

It is widely assumed that psychological distress, depression, and personality disorders are central to temporomandibular pain and dysfunction

Joseph J. Marbach, DDS, is Robert and Susan Carmel Professor in Algesiology, University of Medicine and Dentistry of New Jersey. He was Clinical Professor of Public Health, Division of Sociomedical Science and Department of Psychiatry, Columbia University, and Director of its Pain Research Unit.

Address correspondence to: Dr. Joseph J. Marbach, University of Medicine and Dentistry of New Jersey, Deptment of Psychiatry, 185 South Orange Avenue, Newark, NJ 07103-2714.

This research was supported by National Institute of Dental Research Grant DEO5989.

[Haworth co-indexing entry note]: "Temporomandibular Pain-Dysfunction Syndrome: Evidence for Psychological Etiology?" Marbach, Joseph J. Co-published simultaneously in *Journal of Musculoskeletal Pain* [The Haworth Medical Press, an imprint of The Haworth Press, Inc.] Vol. 4, No. 4, 1996, pp. 155-162; and: *Musculoskeletal Pain Emanating from the Head and Neck: Current Concepts in Diagnosis, Management and Cost Containment* [ed: Murray E. Allen] The Haworth Medical Press, an imprint of The Haworth Press, Inc., 1996, pp. 155-162. Single or multiple copies of this article are available from The Haworth Document Delivery Service [1-800-342-9678, 9:00 a.m. - 5:00 p.m. [EST]. E-mail address: getinfo@haworth.com].

syndrome [TMPDS]. However, this assumes that the same factors influence both the etiology and maintenance of chronic TMPDS. Many treatments are designed to counter a putative etiologic factor without consideration that factors that initiate a disorder may not be the same as those that account for its maintenance, that is, its chronicity. Many widely employed TMPDS treatments are based on clinical lore rather than evidence. Clinicians continue to be trained in unproved but traditionally sanctioned treatments. Such approaches may lead to problems in patient care. Two theories are examined in this paper. The first is that TMPDS is a depressive equivalent or a somatic manifestation of depression. The second theory, posits that TMPDS is a psychophysiological disorder. An interaction between physical and psychological factors are required to produce TMPDS.

Definitions

Musculoskeletal face pain syndromes of unknown etiology are referred to by several names. The term temporomandibular pain dysfunction syndrome, adopted by the International Association for the Study of Pain [IASP], will be employed here (1). The IASP system is intended as a descriptive taxonomy to classify chronic pain syndromes. The IASP criteria for TMPDS are as follows: tenderness in one or more muscles of mastication; besides pain, clicking or popping noise in the temporomandibular joint [TMJ]; and/or restricted mandibular range may be present but are not essential. The TMPDS is characterized by muscle pain associated with localized areas of tenderness on palpation at specific tender points. The TMPDS is distinguished from fibromyalgia chiefly by the site of pain (2).

Extensive research has been conducted on the relationship between life stress and physical health. Various stressors including depression are thought to lead not just to psychopathology but also to physical illness and perhaps even injury proneness. As part of this process the role of stress in the etiology of TMPDS has undergone extensive scrutiny (3-5).

The psychosomatic theory, posits that for certain individuals unresolved conflicts manifest as physical illness. Engle (6) in an influential paper sought to discover a psychoanalytic explanation for pain of unknown origin. He described the "pain-prone patient" as one who suffers from feelings of guilt and depression, for which their chronic pain serves as atonement. Early psychiatric studies of TMPDS patients by Moulton (7) and Schwartz (8) built on these psychosomatic theories. In sum, this theory predicts that cases differ from noncases on traits or long-term personality characteristics. These hypothesized personality traits are thought to find expression as physical illnesses (9).

A second possibility by which personality factors may influence the individual is through intermediate biological mechanisms. Recently, Le-Resche and her colleagues conducted a survey of dentists' knowledge and beliefs about temporomandibular disorders (10). They compared beliefs of a group of "experts" who were selected for extensive contributions to the peer-reviewed literature on TMPDS with a sample of general dentists and dental specialists in the Seattle area. Approximately 85% of the experts surveyed agreed that tooth grinding was often significant in the development of the disorder. A similarly high level of consensus was reached regarding the role of stress and psychological problems as major factors in the development of TMPDS. These findings confirm those of Just et al. (11) who surveyed 1,400 dental practitioners. Thus, despite the skepticism of some (12), the general dental community and also recognized experts in TMPDS believe that stress, psychological problems, and tooth grinding play an important role in the genesis of facial pain.

METHODS

Cases were drawn from the list of a private practitioner. Together 151 women cases and 139 controls entered the study. Eligibility criteria are described elsewhere (13).

Measurement of Potential Personality Risk Factors and Distress

The reliability of the scales measuring personality variables was assessed using Cronbach's (14) alpha, a measure of internal consistency. Reliability coefficients were assessed for cases and controls separately and except for denial [0.52 for cases and 0.44 for controls] were in acceptable range [0.71-0.94 for cases and 0.77-0.90 for controls].

Among the personality variables included is locus of control orientation (15,16). The scales measure the extent to which people believe they exercise control over their lives [internally controlled] or the degree to which they feel their fate is beyond their control and is determined by destiny, chance, or powerful others such as clinicians [externally controlled]. A related personality variable, mastery orientation, was measured with items from Spence-Helmreich's (17) Masculinity and Femininity scales. A measure of denial was constructed from the "blunter" items in the Miller (18) Behavioral Style Scale. The latter scale measures denial as a way of coping with hypothetical life events. Also investigated was Zuckerman's (19) Sensation-Seeking Scale, which may be related to the use of alcohol and drugs. The Marlowe-Crowne (20) Need for Approval Scale was used to measure the need to present oneself in a positive light. A measure of acquiescence derived from the Marlowe-Crowne items was also used.

Nonspecific distress is measured by eight highly correlated symptom scales that, together, measure a phenomenon described as "demoralization" (21). The symptom scales are anxiety, sadness, poor self-esteem, hopelessness-helplessness, dread, confused thinking, psychophysiological symptoms, and perceived physical health. A 27 item measure of demoralization drawn from items in these subscales is used in this paper.

Tooth Grinding

Both cases and controls were asked about current and past tooth grinding (22). They were also asked whether their responses were based on information derived from self-observation or learned from others whom they identified. By this method of questioning, they could provide not only a self-report but also agree or disagree with a dentist or other person regarding their oral habits.

For cases only, a detailed clinical history was recorded that focused specifically on data related physiologically to tooth grinding. This included sites of pain as reported by the patient, presence of morning jaw stiffness, and restricted mandibular range [<35 mm]. The history was followed by a clinical examination that included recording sites of pain elicited by palpation and the determination of maximum mandibular range. Clinical evidence of tooth abrasion was recorded using the notation of Hannson and Nilner (23,24).

RESULTS

Cases do not differ from controls on most of the personality measures. They do show a trend, but toward higher external locus of control perception as measured by the Rotter scale. Thus, the hypothesis that cases of TMPDS differ from controls on important measures of personality characteristics is not supported.

TMPDS cases showed much higher levels of nonspecific psychological distress than did controls. The average score on the distress scale was 1.8 for the women with TMPDS. This represents a score midways between the levels shown by their control group [mean 1.1] and a separate sample of women psychiatric patients [mean of 2.5] with major depression. High scores on distress are just as likely indicators of a response to chronic pain as they are antecedent personality traits.

When comparing cases and controls on grinding rates, cases were not statistically significantly more likely than controls to report ever-grinding, but were significantly less likely than controls to report current grinding [T = 1.98, P < 0.05]. They were also significantly more likely to report that a dentist had told them they grind [T = 2.88, P < 0.01]. These findings are consistent with our central proposition that self-reports of grinding may be influenced by the treating clinician.

Of respondents who report ever-grinding, cases and controls were equally likely to say that they first learned of grinding through a dentist. However, of respondents who report that they never grind, significantly more cases than controls say that a dentist had told them that they ground [T = 4.63, P < 0.0001], again suggesting the strong role of the clinician in influencing patient reports.

DISCUSSION

Contrary to uncontrolled earlier studies, there appears to exist few personality characteristics that distinguish cases from controls. This agrees with several other researchers. Schnurr and colleagues (25) state, "it is somewhat puzzling as to why TMPDS has been considered a psychosomatic disorder. This may, in part, depend on the way in which health care professionals have interacted with the less manageable patients."

The prevailing attitudes of many clinicians that TMPDS cases suffer from a psychological disorder can itself lead to added patient distress (26). Lacking an easily identifiable lesion, people with pain rely on biomedical experts to validate their claims of discomfort through laboratory tests and other medical procedures. Some sources of pain defy explanation by these investigations. When this happens, the person with pain is placed firmly in a situation ripe for pejorative labeling. Consequences of labels follow. The bearer is often discredited in the eyes of others. This, in turn, leads pain sufferers to experience alienation, and self-doubt, while making them vulnerable to potentially inappropriate but "legitimizing" treatments such as TMJ surgery.

Little is firmly known about a disorder's etiology. Where the clinician is motivated to reduce the patient's pain and suffering, there is strong temptation to accept an etiological model that provides a direct treatment strategy: If the pain is caused by tooth grinding, the logical strategy is to initiate treatment such as oral appliances intended to interfere with bruxing. Thus, the temptation to perceive signs of bruxing, even when the evidence is unclear, is undoubtedly strong (27).

Future investigations should test self- and clinician-reported grinding by verifying that certain signs and symptoms of grinding are elevated among reported grinders. It would be useful as well to interview sleep partners of subjects for converging evidence. Laboratory-based studies of experimentally-induced grinding can offer new clues regarding additional signs and symptoms that develop among true grinders. Meanwhile, conclusions regarding the role of grinding in onset or maintenance remain in question. Treatment, assuming tooth grinding as an intermediate variable is, at best, speculative. Especially, given the high cost of treatment for this unproved theory [i.e., intraoral appliances, oral reconstruction] (27) ethical issues also should be considered.

CONCLUSION

Depressed patients are likely to be over-represented as study subjects. Research studies reporting rates of depression or other psychological problems inevitably gather cohorts of chronic pain patients and depression is a risk factor for chronicity. Even in clinical practice, chronic patients are inevitably over-represented, leading even the most conscientious clinician to presume mistakenly that prevalence of depression is unusually high.

It would be premature to conclude that depression is of causal significance in the disorder, even were it shown with more representative samples of TMPDS patients that rates of depression are high compared with general population samples. It is also plausible that depression is a consequence rather than a cause of facial pain or that both are the result of a common tertiary factor. Thus, the comorbidity of depression and facial pain tells one nothing at all about the direction of the causal relationship. As for the question "is there evidence for a psychological etiology of TMPDS," the current answer is a cautious no. Perhaps, future research will change this view. Nevertheless, as more accurate instruments, refined methodologies, and statistical techniques become available evidence for the role of antecedent personality factors recedes in favor of the view that personality abnormalities are consequences of the chronic pain experience.

REFERENCES

1. Merskey H, Bogduk N: Classification of chronic pain. Seattle, IASP Press, 1994, p. 70.

2. Marbach JJ: Is myofascial face pain a regional expression of fibromyalgia? In: Chalmers A, Littlejohn GO, Salit I, Wolfe F (Eds). Fibromyalgia, chronic fatigue syndrome, and repetitive strain injury. New York, Haworth Medical Press, 1995, pp. 93-97.

3. Feinmann C: Psychogenic facial pain: presentation and treatment. J Psychosomatic Research 27: 403-410, 1983.

4. Fine E: Psychological factors associated with non-organic temporomandibular joint dysfunction syndrome. Brit Dent J 131: 402-404, 1971.

5. Eversole LR, Stone CE, Matheson D, et al.: Psychometric profiles and facial pain. Oral Surg Oral Med Oral Path 60: 269-274, 1985.

6. Engle GL: "Psychogenic" pain and the pain-prone patient. Amer J Med 26: 899-918, 1959.

7. Moulton R: Emotional factors in non-organic temporomandibular joint pain. Dent Clinics NA 10: 609-620, 1966.

8. Schwartz L: Disorders of the temporomandibular joint. Philadelphia, W.B. Saunders Co. 1959.

9. Ford C: Chronic Pain Syndrome, The somatizing disorders: illness a way of life. New York, Elsevier 1983.

10. LeResche L, Truelove EL, Dworkin SF: Temporomandibular disorders: a survey of dentists' knowledge and beliefs. J Amer dent Assoc 124: 91-106, 1993.

11. Just JK, Perry HT, Greene CS: Treating TM disorders: a survey on diagnosis, etiology, and management. J Amer dent Assoc 122: 55-60 1991.

12. Lund JP: Review and commentary (A) Basic Sciences. Research Diagnostic criteria of temporomandibular disorders. J Cranio Dis: Facial & Oral Pain 6: 346-350 1993.

13. Marbach JJ, Lennon MC, Dohrenwend BP: Candidate risk factors for temporomandibular pain and dysfunction syndrome: psychosocial, health behavior, physical illness and injury. Pain 34:139-151, 1988.

14. Cronbach LJ: Coefficient alpha and the internal structure of tests. J Psychometrika 16: 297-334, 1951.

15. Rotter JB: Generalized expectancies of internal versus external control of reinforcement. Psych Mono 80, 1966.

16. Levenson H: Multidimensional locus of control in psychiatric patients. J Consulting Clin Psych 4: 397-404, 1973.

17. Spence JT, Helmreich R: Masculinity and Femininity: Their Psychological Dimensions. Correlates, and Antecedents. Austin, University of Texas Press, 1978.

18. Miller SM: When is a little information a dangerous thing? Coping with stressful events by monitoring vs. blunting. In: Levine, S., Ursin, H., eds. Coping and Health: Proceedings of a NATO Conference. New York, Plenum Press, 1980.

19. Zuckerman M: Dimensions of sensation seeking. J Consulting Clin Psych 36: 45-52, 1971.

20. Crowne DP, Marlowe D: The Approval Motive: Studies in Evaluative Dependence. New York, Wiley, 1964.

21. Dohrenwend BP, Shrout PE, Egri G, et al.: Measures of nonspecific psychological distress and other dimensions of psychopathology in the general population. Arch Gen Psychiat 37: 1229-1236, 1980.

22. Marbach JJ, Raphael KG, Dohrenwend BP, et al.: The validity of tooth grinding measures: etiology of pain dysfunction syndrome revisited. J Amer dent Assoc 120: 327-333, 1990.

23. Hannson T, Nilner M: A study of the occurrence of symptoms of diseases of the temporomandibular joint masticatory musculature and related structures. J Oral Rehab 2: 313-324, 1975.

24. Rugh JD, Harlan J: Nocturnal bruxism and temporomandibular disorders. In: Jankovic J, Tolosa E (Eds). Advances in neurology: facial dyskinesias. New York, Raven Press 49: 329-341, 1988.

25. Schnurr RF, Brooke RI, Rollman GB: Psychosocial correlates of temporomandibular joint pain and dysfunction. Pain 42: 153-165, 1990.

26. Marbach JJ, Lennon MC, Link BG, et al.: Losing face: sources of stigma as perceived by chronic facial pain patients. J Behav Med 13: 583-604, 1990.

27. Dao TTT, Lavigne GJ, Charbonneau A, et al.: The efficacy of oral splints in the treatment of myofascial pain of the jaw muscles: a controlled clinical trial. Pain 56: 85-94, 1994.

Guarded Movements:
Development of Chronicity

Chris J. Main
Paul J. Watson

SUMMARY. Despite increasing advances in medical technology, the cost of musculoskeletal incapacity, particularly low-back pain, in terms of sickness benefits, invalidity benefits and associated allowances has led to a fundamental reconsideration of the nature of chronic incapacity. Recent reports from the United Kingdom and the United States of America, in their recommendations for a comprehensive multidisciplinary assessment for patients still symptomatic at six weeks, are based on the clear assumption that a significant proportion of chronic incapacity is preventable. Such a proposition represents a fundamental challenge to much of current medical practice. *[Article copies available from The Haworth Document Delivery Service: 1-800-342-9678. E-mail address: getinfo@haworth.com]*

Chris J. Main, MA [Hons], MPhil, PhD, FSPsS, is Associate Professor, University of Manchester, and Research Director, Manchester and Salford Back Pain Centre. He is Associate Editor of SPINE, and is Convenor of the International Association for the Study of Pain Task Force on Development of a Curriculum on Pain for Psychologists.

Paul J. Watson, BSc [Hons], MSc, MCSP is Research Physiotherapist, Rheumatic Diseases Centre, University of Manchester, Manchester, UK, and Lecturer in Physiotherapy and Pain Management, Manchester School of Physiotherapy, Manchester, UK.

Address correspondence to: Dr. Chris J. Main, Department Behavioural Medicine, Hope Hospital, Clinical Sciences Building, Eccles Old Road, Salford/Manchester, M68HD UK.

The authors would like to acknowledge Kerry Booker.

[Haworth co-indexing entry note]: "Guarded Movements: Development of Chronicity." Main, Chris J., and Paul J. Watson. Co-published simultaneously in *Journal of Musculoskeletal Pain* [The Haworth Medical Press, an imprint of The Haworth Press, Inc.] Vol. 4, No. 4, 1996, pp. 163-170; and: *Musculoskeletal Pain Emanating from the Head and Neck: Current Concepts in Diagnosis, Management and Cost Containment* [ed: Murray E. Allen] The Haworth Medical Press, an imprint of The Haworth Press, Inc., 1996, pp. 163-170. Single or multiple copies of this article are available from The Haworth Document Delivery Service [1-800-342-9678, 9:00 a.m. - 5:00 p.m. [EST]. E-mail address: getinfo@haworth.com].

163

CLINICAL MODELS OF ILLNESS AND INCAPACITY

There has been an increasing recognition that an adequate understanding of illness, and particularly of chronic incapacity requires a broader perspective than the traditional disease model. Waddell (1) in the Glasgow Illness model identified distress, pain behavior and social factors as contributory to patients' overall level of disability. The biopsychosocial model, as it came to be known, was further refined by the incorporation of beliefs about pain into a dynamic model addressing the transition from acute to chronic incapacity (2). The model will be discussed in more detail below.

Nature of Psychological Factors

During the last 15 years, the role of psychological factors in the genesis and maintenance of pain problems has been increasingly recognized. Early research into personality traits and identifiable psychiatric illness has been followed by investigation of more specific psychological characteristics such as psychological distress, pain behavior, beliefs about pain and pain coping strategies. A range of psychometric tests, behavioral measures and more general tools assessing function or impact of pain have been developed both for the assessment of pain and the investigation of specific psychological dimensions. A detailed discussion of the use and interpretation of such tests is far beyond the remit of this article, but a number of tests will be mentioned for illustrative purposes.

The patient's pain may be assessed by means of a questionnaire such as the Short-Form McGill Pain Questionnaire [MPQ] (3). Although the test has been widely used as a research tool and incorporates a number of different scoring mechanisms, clinically it is used primarily to distinguish between sensory and emotional components of pain by an analysis of pain vocabulary. It has been claimed that emotional content can also be identified using the Pain Drawing Test, but a recent study (4) has demonstrated that although patients with clearly abnormal pain drawings are almost always distressed, 50% of distressed patients produce normal pain drawings.

The Minnesota Multiphasic Personality Inventory [MMPI and MMPI-2] (5) have been widely used, particularly in North America, for the assessment of personality traits. While the historical pedigree of the MMPI is undeniable, its specific value for clinical assessment has recently been questioned (6). Simpler measures of distress [comprising assessment of somatic awareness and depressive symptomatology] such as the Distress Risk Assessment Method [DRAM] (7), are more sharply focused and certainly more practical, but while the DRAM may be useful as the basis of an assessment system, it would need additional psychological dimensions to offer more than a psychological screen or classification. A wide range of tests is available for the assessment of attitudes or beliefs about pain and specific coping strategies. Beliefs about pain locus of control can be assessed using one of several questionnaires, but specific fears about hurting and harming may turn out to be more discriminating. The Fear-Avoidance Beliefs Questionnaire [FABQ] (2) is one such questionnaire which has been recently developed. A recent study (8) has shown that fear of movement may have a major impact on behavioral performance. This topic would seem to merit further investigation. Specific cognitive coping strategies should also be assessed. The most widely used questionnaire is the Coping Strategies Questionnaire [CSQ] (9) which consists of a set of scales assessing positive [or potentially effective] coping strategies and negative [or ineffective] coping strategies. Several studies have shown that negative or ineffective coping strategies such as catastrophising ["fearing the worst"] are associated with higher levels of self-reported disability or adjustment.

Where it is possible to conduct serial assessment, aspects of pain behavior such as grimacing or guarding may be rated using direct observational methods with specially designed rating scales for the assessment of pain behaviors, but more accurate and sophisticated tools such as the Behavioral Observation Test (10) are also available. It consists of a standardized 10-minute video-taped assessment during which a number of specific pain behaviors are rated. The test, however, requires careful training for use and videotaped assessment often is not a practical possibility.

Predictors of Chronic Incapacity

Although there are significant methodological problems in the definition of recurrence and chronicity, a number of studies have attempted to identify predictors of chronicity. In the clinical assessment of low-back pain, the lack of a simple relationship between physical signs and resulting incapacity is well recognized and different sorts of factors have been adduced to explain the apparent mismatch. Recent clinical studies into the outcome of treatment for low-pain have, however, offered a more specific evaluation of the role of different sorts of psychological variables in the prediction of chronic incapacity [as determined by self-reported disability] than is currently available in most occupational studies. The findings of such studies for our understanding of the nature and development of chronic incapacity may have relevance also to secondary prevention in occupational settings and so some of these studies will now be reviewed.

In a recent study of patients attending a department of orthopaedic surgery with back pain, it was found that psychological characteristics in terms of depressive and somatic symptoms were strongly associated with outcome of treatment, in terms of pain and disability two years later (7). Such characteristics have been found similarly predictive of outcome of treatment of acute low-back pain, both immediately following treatment and at one year follow-up (Roberts et al., unpublished observation). Finally in a one year follow-up of patients with back pain attending for osteopathic treatment, cognitive factors [specifically negative or inappropriate coping strategies] were found to be by far the most powerful predictors of outcome; particularly in the sub-group of patients with acute back pain in which it was possible to explain 47% of variance in outcome from negative cognitive coping strategies alone (11).

Conclusion of Conceptual Overview

Clinical studies have identified a range of predictors of outcome of treatment and rehabilitation. In general psychological factors seem to be much more important determinants of outcome than physical or demographic factors. Studies of outcome of treatment for acute back pain have identified levels of distress and pain coping strategies as particularly powerful determinants of future incapacity. Most of the research reported above has used either cross-sectional designs or prospective cohort analysis. Recently in our laboratories we have been investigating the specific interaction between physical and psychological factors in patients presenting with musculoskeletal pain problems, particularly low-back pain using surface electromyography [sEMG]. The salient features of the research program will now be outlined.

PSYCHOPHYSIOLOGICAL MECHANISMS OF CHRONICITY

Establishment of the Research Laboratory

Since international standards vary considerably regarding the licensing of clinical assessment systems, it was necessary initially to satisfy ourselves of the accuracy of the data capture system. Although the primary consideration is, of course, patient safety, we needed a research tool capable of a higher degree of precision than that usually required by clinicians. A new temperature and humidity controlled laboratory was developed and following some months of equipment validation, a satisfactory degree of accuracy in data capture was demonstrated. A critical evaluation of different types of electrodes was also carried out.

Standardization of Skin Preparation and Electrode Placements

Particular attention was paid to the minimization of "noise" between skin and electrode, and electrodes were placed over the body of the muscle, in the direction of the muscle fibers. Choice of muscle scanning sites was investigated following Cram (12), but the overall principal choice of site was based on the identification of muscles associated with particular movements rather than on concepts of comprehensiveness of a wide sampling of different spinal levels. For the purpose of the initial set of studies, six principal sites at three levels were chosen for analysis of dynamic activity: L1/2, L4/5 and T10. At each site bilateral assessment was made by placing pairs of electrodes equidistant from the mid-point of the spine. For the purpose of sEMG patterning during static postural assessment [sitting and standing], six sites were analysed bilaterally and were simultaneously monitored. The results presented will be those based on bilateral sEMG activity at levels L1/2 and L4/5 during a 15 second flexion and re-extension cycle. The precise parameters investigated will be described below.

Standardization of Posture During Surface
Electromyography Assessment

A series of experiments were conducted to establish the reliability and discriminative validity of these sEMG measures used.

Experiment one. The sEMG activity at the sites above in 70 patients with chronic low-back pain [CLBP] were compared with 20 healthy controls drawn from Healthcare and University populations. Inclusion criteria into the control group were: never having consulted for back pain, no history of back pain in the previous 12 months, no history of chronic pelvic or abdominal pain. The results demonstrated that there were significant differences in the dynamic activities monitored between the two groups.

Experiment two. Eleven CLBP patients were assessed repeatedly over a four week period to identify the intra- and inter-test reliability of the measures. Those measures that were reliable were used to assess the outcome from a pain management program in experiment three.

Experiment three. The relationships among the observed dynamic sEMG abnormalities, ranges of spinal movement, pain report, fear avoidance and self-efficacy beliefs were investigated. Data was gathered before and after a pain management program and the changes as a result of the program were assessed. The results demonstrated no relationship between range of lumbar motion, pain intensity [measured on the MPQ] and abnormalities of muscle action on sEMG. There was a significant correlation, however, between fear avoidance beliefs and abnormalities of muscle action prior to the pain management program. Following the pain management program there were significant correlations between changes in the muscular abnormalities and changes in fear avoidance beliefs as well as between changes in self-efficacy beliefs and changes in muscular abnormalities.

Experiment four. A group of fourteen CLBP patients and a group of age and sex matched healthy controls underwent a tonic pain provocation test using a cold-pressor test [CPT]. The sEMG activity at lumbar paraspinal and upper trapezius muscle sites were monitored during five stages: baseline, hand in cold water, hand out of cold water, hand in iced water [CPT] and hand out of iced water. Each phase lasted for three minutes. The results demonstrated significant differences in the responses at the two sites during the CPT. Healthy control subjects demonstrated a reflex increase in sEMG in the upper trapezius. The CLBP patients demonstrated increased activity in the lumbar region and an absence of the reflex activity at the trapezius site.

Conclusions of Surface Electromyography Dynamic Activity

1. It has been possible to identify discrete patterns of sEMG activity which distinguish asymptomatic normals from patients with chronic low-back pain.
2. These patterns appear to be accurate and reliable.
3. Results from the cold-presser test experiment raise the possibility that following injury, or a significant painful episode, some people develop persistent abnormalities in muscle electrical activity suggestive of a persistent physiological abnormality around the painful site.
4. The extent to which these abnormalities are mediated by fears of hurting and harming is not yet entirely clear, but changes in sEMG patterns towards the normal following pain management are associated with reductions in fear of hurting and harming and increased self-efficacy beliefs.
5. Since patients are not normally aware of these changes in electrical activity, we may be observing an unconsciously learned conditioned emotional response following injury.
6. The initial results of our investigations offer an explanation for the development of chronic musculoskeletal pain. The next logical step would be to examine prospectively recently injured patients, such as those following a discrete injury such as whiplash-associated disorder [WAD] (13).

DISCUSSION AND CONCLUSIONS

In general the individual's response to injury and beliefs about work have not been considered as major risk factors in the development of chronicity. On the basis of the clinical studies reviewed, it would seem essential to include assessment of levels of distress, beliefs about pain, coping strategies and perception of work routinely if unnecessary chronicity is to be prevented.

Investigations into the early development of chronicity have consisted of primary prevention programs, such as industrial back schools, or identification of dangers in the work environment. Preventative efforts, derived from an ergonomic and biomechanical perspective have tended to focus on approaches such as training in lifting and handling techniques. Clinical studies, however, have until recently relied almost exclusively on studies of chronic pain patients. Recent studies of patients with acute back pain, however, have demonstrated that psychological features at the time of injury or soon thereafter have a powerful influence on outcome of treatment and the development of chronic incapacity. These findings are consistent with preliminary laboratory studies into the characteristics and mechanisms of chronicity revealed in the investigation of guarded movements using sEMG from paraspinal musculature. It would appear that future research might usefully be directed at secondary prevention [in addition to tertiary rehabilitation] with the development of accurate assessment protocols capable of accurately documenting outcome of treatment and facilitating better selection of patients with treatment protocols based on identified patient need.

REFERENCES

1. Waddell G, McCulloch JA, Kummel E, Main CJ: Symptoms and signs: physical disease or illness behaviour. BMJ 289: 739-741, 1984.

2. Waddell G, Somerville D, Henderson I, Newton M, Main CJ: A fear avoidance beliefs questionnaire (FABQ) and the role of fear avoidance beliefs in chronic low back pain and disability. Pain 52: 157-168, 1993.

3. Melzack R: The short form McGill Pain Questionnaire. Pain 30: 191-197, 1987.

4. Parker H, Wood PLR, Main CJ: The use of the pain drawing as a screening measure to predict psychological distress in chronic low back pain. Spine 20(2): 236-243, 1995.

5. Butcher JN, Dahlstrom WG, Graham JR, Tellegren A, Kaemmer B: Manual for the administration and scoring. Multiphasic Personality Inventory 2: MMPI-2 University of Minnesota Press, 1989.

6. Main CJ, Spanswick CC: Personality assessment and the MMPI. 50 years on: Do we still need our security blanket? Pain Forum 4: 60-66, 1995.

7. Main CJ, Wood PLR, Hollis S, Spanswick CC, Waddell G: The distress assessment method: A simple patient classification to identify distress and evaluate risk of poor outcome. Spine 17(1): 42-50, 1992.

8. Vlaeyen JWS, Kole-Snijders AJ, Boeren RGB, van Eek H: Fear of movement/(re)injury in chronic low back pain and its relation to behavioural performance. Pain 62: 363-372, 1995.

9. Rosenstiel AK, Keefe FJ: The use of coping strategies in chronic low back pain patients: Relationship to patient characteristics and current adjustments. Pain 17: 33-34, 1983.

10. Keefe FJ, Hill RW: An objective approach to quantifying pain behaviour and gait patterns in low back pain patients. Pain 21: 153-161, 1985.

11. Burton AK, Tillotson MK, Main CJ, Hollis S: "Psychosocial predictors of outcome in acute and sub-chronic low back trouble." Spine 20:722-728, 1995.

12. Cram JR: Clinic EMG surface recordings Vol 2. Clinical Resources, Nevada City, 1990.

13. Spitzer WO, et al.: Scientific Monograph of the Quebec Task Force on Whiplash Associated Disorders: Redefining "Whiplash and its management." Spine 20: (Supplement 8S) 1s-73s, 1995.

Index

Page numbers followed by "t" denote tables and "f" denote figures.

Abbreviated Injury Scale, velocity
    change and, 31
Abel, M.S., 83
Acceleration/deceleration. *See* Peak
    acceleration; Velocity change
Acceleration peak, 25
Accident neurosis, 44
Accidents, vehicular. *See* Occupant
    dynamics; Vehicular
    collisions
Affective arousal, 151. *See also*
    Attention
Age. *See also* Osteoarthritis
    blunt trauma injuries and, 64
    effects of versus injury, 64,77
Aljinovic, M., 6
Alker, G.J., 72
Allen, L., 87,89
Allen, M.E., xiii,16
Allen, M.J., 41
American Dental Association, 137
American Psychiatric Association,
    56
Amusement park bumper car study,
    35-36
Analgesics, 128-129
Anderson, R.D., 14,15,30,31,
    35,41,43
Anesthesia, controlled diagnostic
    (block), 88-89
Anthropomorphic dummies
    biofidelity lacking in, 12-13,31
    Hybrid II, 40
    Hybrid III, 12-13

Anxiety, 141-142
Aprill, C., 77,84,85,86,87,89
Arntz, A., 150
Assendelft, W.J.J., 128
Assessment. *See* Diagnosis
Atkinson, J.H., 149
Atlanto-axial joint injury, 68
Atlanto-occipital joint injury,
    68,88,89
Attention, 50,51,151
Attribution theory (locus of control),
    148-149
Aufdermaur, M., 63
Australia, 42
    Australian Neuromuscular
        Research Institute, 61-77
    University of Newcastle, 81-91
Automobile design, 15-16
Autopsy studies. *See also* Cervical
    spinal injury studies
    serial sagittal sectioning
        technique, 72-73
    of spinal trauma as compared
        with radiography, 61-77
Avoidance of activity,
    150-151,163-169

Bailey, M., 14,15,25,29,35
Bailey, Mark, 21-37
Baker Materials Engineering Ltd.,
    11-18
Balance impairment, 105-111
Balcerak, J.C., 12,16,17

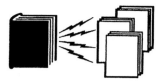

Haworth
DOCUMENT DELIVERY
SERVICE

This valuable service provides a single-article order form for any article from a Haworth journal.

- *Time Saving:* No running around from library to library to find a specific article.
- *Cost Effective:* All costs are kept down to a minimum.
- *Fast Delivery:* Choose from several options, including same-day FAX.
- *No Copyright Hassles:* You will be supplied by the original publisher.
- *Easy Payment:* Choose from several easy payment methods.

Open Accounts Welcome for . . .
- Library Interlibrary Loan Departments
- Library Network/Consortia Wishing to Provide Single-Article Services
- Indexing/Abstracting Services with Single Article Provision Services
- Document Provision Brokers and Freelance Information Service Providers

---

MAIL or *FAX* THIS ENTIRE ORDER FORM TO:

Haworth Document Delivery Service
The Haworth Press, Inc.
10 Alice Street
Binghamton, NY 13904-1580

or FAX: 1-800-895-0582
or CALL: 1-800-342-9678
9am-5pm EST

PLEASE SEND ME PHOTOCOPIES OF THE FOLLOWING SINGLE ARTICLES:
1) Journal Title: _____

    Vol/Issue/Year: _____Starting & Ending Pages: _____
Article Title: _____

2) Journal Title: _____

    Vol/Issue/Year: _____Starting & Ending Pages: _____
Article Title: _____

3) Journal Title: _____

    Vol/Issue/Year: _____Starting & Ending Pages: _____
Article Title: _____

4) Journal Title: _____

    Vol/Issue/Year: _____Starting & Ending Pages: _____
Article Title: _____

(See other side for Costs and Payment Information)

COSTS: Please figure your cost to order quality copies of an article.

1. Set-up charge per article: $8.00
   ($8.00 × number of separate articles)   _____
2. Photocopying charge for each article:
   1-10 pages: $1.00   _____

   11-19 pages: $3.00   _____

   20-29 pages: $5.00   _____

   30+ pages: $2.00/10 pages   _____
3. Flexicover (optional): $2.00/article   _____
4. Postage & Handling: US: $1.00 for the first article/
   $.50 each additional article   _____

   Federal Express: $25.00   _____

   Outside US: $2.00 for first article/
   $.50 each additional article_____
5. Same-day FAX service: $.35 per page   _____

GRAND TOTAL: _____

METHOD OF PAYMENT: (please check one)

❑ Check enclosed   ❑ Please ship and bill. PO # _____
(sorry we can ship and bill to bookstores only! All others must pre-pay)

❑ Charge to my credit card: ❑ Visa; ❑ MasterCard; ❑ Discover;
❑ American Express;

Account Number:_____ Expiration date:_____

Signature: ✗_____

Name: _____ Institution: _____

Address: _____

_____

City: _____ State:_____ Zip:_____

Phone Number: _____ FAX Number: _____

MAIL or *FAX* THIS ENTIRE ORDER FORM TO:

Haworth Document Delivery Service	**or FAX:** 1-800-895-0582
The Haworth Press, Inc.	**or CALL:** 1-800-342-9678
10 Alice Street	9am-5pm EST)
Binghamton, NY 13904-1580	